Kundalini Yoga

KUNDALINI YOGA:
THE MYSTERIES
OF THE FIRE

by

Samael Aun Weor

GLORIAN

Kundalini Yoga: The Mysteries of Fire
A Glorian Book / 2012

Originally published in Spanish as "Los Misterios del
Fuego" (1955).

Print: 978-1-934206-10-2
Ebook: 978-1-934206-47-8

Glorian Publishing is a non-profit organization. All
proceeds go to further the distribution of these books.
For more information, visit our websites.

gnosticteachings.org

Contents

In the Vestibule of Wisdom

Beloved disciple,

Many books have been written about Oriental yoga. Yoga means "union with God." All the books that were written about Oriental yoga before now are antiquated for the new era of Aquarius, which began the fourth of February 1962, between the hours of two and three in the afternoon.

This book entitled *Kundalini Yoga* is for the new Aquarian era. Through this book we teach our disciples a practical religion. All religions teach us unbreakable dogmas in which we are supposed to believe, even when their truths cannot be seen with eyes of the flesh. Regarding the former statement, we, the Gnostics, are a little different. We teach the human being to see, hear, touch, and perceive all of the things from beyond the grave, the divine mysteries, the ineffable things, etc.

We sustain that human beings have a sixth sense, and that through this sixth sense they can see the angels and converse with them.

We asseverate that human beings have a seventh sense called "intuition." Thus, when human beings awaken that seventh sense they can know the great mysteries of life and death. Then they do not need to study these mysteries in any book. So, beloved reader, this book is for that purpose.

You will find terrific secrets within this book, secrets that never in the history of life were published.

We respect all religions profoundly. Not only do we respect them, but moreover, we teach our disciples how to see, hear, touch, and perceive the essential truths that all religions teach in their sacred books.

Therefore, this book that you have in your hands is a book of terrific secrets that have never been published before. You can develop your occult powers to see, hear, touch and perceive the Angels, Archangels, Seraphim, Potentates, Virtues, etc. You can attain yoga—union with God—with this book.

The Holy Bible discloses great truths; thus, we read within the Bible how the prophets of God had the power to talk with the angels.

This book that you have in your hands belongs to the Gnostic Christian Universal Church; read it, study it, and meditate on it. This is the yoga of the new era of Aquarius.

You will find a glossary at the end of this book with the explanation of the meaning of many words that you may not know. Therefore, search in the glossary for the meaning of each word that you do not know [additional words can be found online at GnosticTeachings.org]

We are entering the ethereal world, where the human being has to conquer the fifth element of nature, the ether. The ethereal world (fourth dimension) has to be the conquest of the Aryan Race [The term Aryan refers to all the people of this planet, not one group. Read "Aryan" in the glossary on page 146]. Gross material- ism must fall wounded before the majesty of the ether. This book is for those who indeed want to transform themselves into angels.

Every planet gives birth to seven root races; thereafter it dies. Our planet Earth already gave birth to five root races; two more root races are needed. There are seven elements of nature.

The first root race lived in the polar cap of the north and conquered the fire.

The second root race, after having fought against the tempestuous atmosphere of the air from the second continent, the Hyperborean continent, finally attained the conquest of the air and adapted themselves to its environment.

The third root race lived in Lemuria, fighting against the tempestuous seas, and was removed by incessant seaquakes. The third root race conquered the water.

The fourth root race lived in the continent of Atlantis within an aqueous

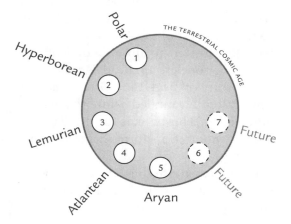

atmosphere. Human beings breathed though gills; but a total transformation happened in the human physiognomy with the Deluge: the human being developed his lungs and adapted himself to the new atmosphere. Then the human being perceived the physical world with his sight and he conquered the element earth.

Presently we are in the Aryan Root Race, which populates the five continents of the world. The triumph of this root race has not yet been achieved. The Aryan Root Race will conquer the ether. Atomic investigations will take the human being to the conquest of ether.

Interplanetary ships occupied by people from other worlds, from different planets of the solar system, will come to the Earth. These types of ships are owned by any advanced humanity from any of the planets of space. However, these cosmic ships have not been delivered to this terrestrial humanity for the simple fact that they will use them in order to perpetrate in other planets the same barbarian invasions that they accomplished here in their historical conquests.

The people from any of the planets of this solar system are already very advanced and they know very well the state of barbarism in which we, the inhabitants of Earth, are found. Nevertheless, in the new era of Aquarius, the inhabitants of the different worlds of the solar system will establish official contact with our planet Earth.

Human beings from other humanities, like Venus, Mars, Mercury, etc., will come in interplanetary ships and many people will go aboard those ships to know the different planets of the solar system. Those advanced humanities will teach the human being how to build those interplanetary ships. This is how the official science will be fulminated and human pride will be wounded to death by the advanced humanities from this solar system.

In the new Aquarian era, the Aryan Root Race will conquer the interplanetary ether, and cosmic trips to other planets will become routine. Cultural and commercial interaction will be established with all of the solar system; thus, as a consequence, the human being will elevate himself to a high cultural level.

Later on, the Sixth Root Race that will inhabit the continent of Antarctica will conquer the Astral Light.

The Seventh Root Race will conquer the Cosmic Mind; then, the human being will elevate himself to the angelic kingdom.

Nonetheless, I tell you, beloved reader, that with this book that you have in your hands, right now, you can transform into a terrific divine angel, if that is what you want. What is important is for you to practice the terrific divine science which we are delivering to you in this book.

May peace be with this entire humanity.

Samael Aun Weor

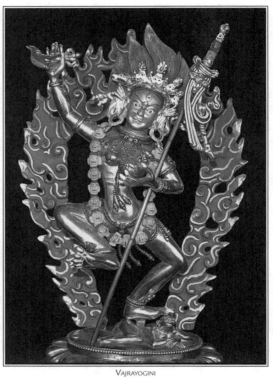

VAJRAYOGINI

Chapter 1

The Universal Fire

1. Maha-Kundalini is Fohat.

2. Maha-Kundalini is the universal fire of life.

3. The universal fire has seven degrees of power.

4. Oh Devi Kundalini! You are the fire of the seven Laya centers of the universe.

5. The seven Laya centers of the universe are the seven degrees of power of the fire.

6. There are seven churches in the Chaos where the seven planetary Logoi officiate.

7. These seven churches are also within the spinal medulla of the human being.

8. The seven planetary Logoi officiated in their seven temples in the dawn of life.

9. The seven saints practiced the rituals of Maha-Kundalini within the sacred

precinct of their temples in the dawn of the Mahamanvantara.

10. The material universe did not exist.

11. The universe solely existed within the mind of the gods.

12. Nonetheless, for the gods, the universe was ideal and objective, simultaneously.

13. The universe was; yet, it did not exist.

14. The universe "is;" yet, it does not exist within the bosom of the Absolute.

15. To be is better than to exist.

16. The seven saints fecundated the chaotic matter so that universal life could emerge.

17. Devi Kundalini has seven degrees of power.

18. There are seven serpents: two groups of three, plus the sublime coronation of the seventh tongue of fire that unites us with the One, with the Law, with the Father.

19. These seven degrees of power of the fire differentiated the chaotic matter in seven states of matter upon which the perceptions of our seven senses are based.

20. The seven igneous serpents of each of the planetary Logoi fecundated the chaotic matter so that life could emerge.

21. Sattva, Rajas, and Tamas (harmony, emotion, and inertness)* were in a perfect, Nirvanic equilibrium before the dawning of the aurora of the Mahamanvantara.

22. The fire put the cosmic scale in motion.

23. Sattva, Rajas, and Tamas became unbalanced; thus, this is how the Mahamanvantara dawned.

24. The yogi/yogini must liberate their Self from Sattva, Rajas, and Tamas in order to gain the right to enter into the Absolute.

25. Sattva, Rajas, and Tamas will be in perfect equilibrium again at the end of the Mahamanvantara; thus, the universe will sleep again within the profound bosom of the Absolute, within the supreme Parabrahman, the Nameless.

* Known in Sanskrit as the Gunas.

26. The universe will sleep for seven eternities, until Maha-Kundalini awakens it again to activity.

27. The Chaos is the raw matter of the Great Work.

28. The Chaos is the Mulaprakriti, the primordial matter.

29. Mulaprakriti is Christonic semen, from which the universe emerged.

30. We have Mulaprakriti in our sexual organs, and thence it springs up life.

31. We see seven sacred vessels filled with Christonic semen upon the altars of the temples of the seven planetary Logoi.

32. That is the sacred symbol of Mulaprakriti.

33. Those are the primordial waters of life.

34. The water is the habitat of fire.

35. The one who wastes the water also wastes the fire and remains in darkness.

36. The seven saints fecundated the Christonic semen of the universe so that life could sprout.

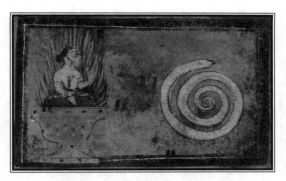

37. The yogi/yogini has to fecundate his primordial waters, his Christonic semen, with the grandiose power of Devi Kundalini.

38. Kundalini is the spouse of Shiva, the Innermost, the Purusha.

39. Kundalini is the spirit of electricity.

40. Electricity is the sexual power of Maha-Kundalini.

41. Kundalini is coiled within the chakra Muladhara.

42. Kundalini is the serpent whose tail is coiled three and a half times.

43. When Kundalini awakens, it hisses as the serpents hisses.

44. The Prana, the Buddhi, the Indriyas, the Ahamkara, the mind, the seven

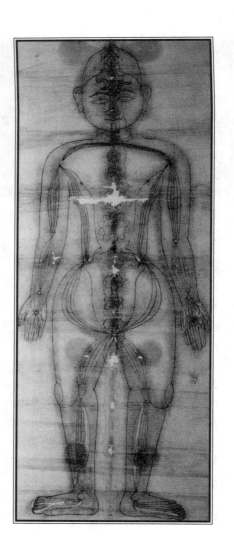

elements of nature, the nerves, are in their totality products of Kundalini.

45. Kundalini is intimately related with the Prana that circulates throughout the 72,000 nadis or Astral conduits that nourish the chakras.

46. The chakras are connected with the mind.

47. Yogi and yogini have to christify their mind.

48. Prana is life, and it circulates throughout all of our organs.

49. Prana circulates throughout all of our nadis and vital canals.

50. All of the 72,000 nadis of our organism have their fundamental base in the nadi Kanda.

51. The nadi Kanda is situated between the sexual organs and the anus.

52. The Kanda collects all of the sexual energy that circulates throughout the 72,000 canals of our organism.

53. The sexual energy is Prana, life.

54. The Angel Aroch (angel of power) taught us the pranava **Kandil, Bandil, R** for the awakening of Devi Kundalini.

55. These mantras act over the Kanda, reinforcing the vibration of Prana.

56. Thus, the spouse of Shiva, who is coiled in the chakra Muladhara, is awakened when Prana is reinforced.

57. The correctly chanted pronunciation of this pranava is as follows:

58. ***KAN dil... BAN dil... Rrrrrrrrrr...***

59. KAN is pronounced aloud. DIL is pronounced with a low voice.

60. BAN is pronounced aloud. DIL is pronounced with a low voice.

61. The letter R has to be rolled and acutely pronounced, imitating the sound produced by the rattles of the rattlesnake.

62. This is how the Prana is reinforced, so that from the Kanda—where the Shushumna nadi and the chakra Muladhara are joined—Devi Kundalini awakens.

63. The Kanda is precisely situated in the same point where the nadi Shushumna and the chakra Muladhara join.

64. This is why the pranava of the Angel Aroch acts so intensely over the Kundalini.

65. The Kanda nourishes itself with the sexual organs.

66. The Kanda has its physiological correspondence in the "cauda equina" of the spinal medulla.

67. The spinal medulla begins in the spinal bulbar region (this refers to the medulla oblongata, which looks like a swelling, or bulb, at the top of the spinal cord), and ends in the cauda equina (because of their appearance, the obliquely coursing fine nerve roots or nerve fibers are named the cauda equina, a Latin term for "horse's tail"), that form the inferior extreme of the spinal medulla.

68. Prana is sexual.

69. The sexual energy is solar.

70. The solar energy is Christic.

71. Prana is Christic.

72. The Cosmic Christ is the Solar Logos.

73. The solar energy comes from the Cosmic Christ.

74. The Christic Prana makes the spike of wheat grow; thus, the Christic substance—ready to be devoured—remains enclosed within the grain.

75. The water from the mountain glaciers penetrates within the stump to ripen the grape, within which the whole life, the whole Prana from the Sun-Christ, remains enclosed.

76. This is why the bread and the wine symbolize the flesh and blood of the martyr of Calvary.

77. All vegetables evolve with the potent force of the Solar Logos.

78. All food disarranges itself into billions of solar corpuscular energies within our organic laboratory.

79. These solar corpuscular energies are called vitamins by the men of science.

80. The best of the radiant force of the Sun remains enclosed within our sexual glands.

81. The very aroma of the Sun, the most powerful solar atoms, form that semi-solid, semi-liquid substance that is called Christonic semen or Mulaprakriti.

82. Mulaprakriti is the Cosmic Christ in substance.

83. Therefore, the entire power of Devi Kundalini is within our Christonic semen.

84. Whosoever wants to awaken Devi Kundalini has to be absolutely chaste.

85. Whosoever wants to awaken Devi Kundalini has to know how to wisely control the sexual forces.

86. The wise control of the sexual energies is called sexual magic.

87. Not a single yogi/yogini can totally Christify their Self without sexual magic.

88. The Kanda is found situated within the chakra Muladhara.

89. The chakra Muladhara has four resplendent petals.

90. The Kanda has the shape of an egg.

91. The Kanda nourishes itself with the Cosmic Christ.

92. When the Kundalini awakens, it rises throughout the spinal medulla.

93. The Brahmanadi or "canalis centralis" within which the Kundalini ascends

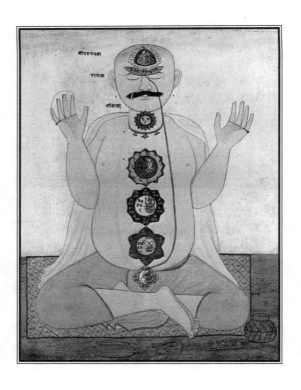

is throughout the length of the spinal medulla.

94. Our planet Earth also has its spinal column.

95. The spinal column of our planet earth is Mount Meru, situated in the Himalayas.

96. The chakra Muladhara is the abode of Devi Kundalini.

97. The chakra Muladhara is found situated at the very root of our sexual organs.

98. Therefore, the chakra Muladhara is totally sexual and can be opened only with sexual magic.

99. Sexual magic has always been taught in secrecy within the secret schools of Oriental yoga.

100. In our next chapters, we will teach to our disciples the complete sexual magic of India and Tibet, just as it has always been taught in the secret schools.

101. Now, it is necessary for our disciples to chant daily the pranava of the Angel Aroch.

102. It is urgent to vocalize daily these mantras for one hour.

103. This is how we will reinforce the Prana, by intensely acting over the Kanda, to awaken the spouse of Shiva, Devi Kundalini.

104. Maha-Kundalini underlies in all organic and inorganic matter and is the cause of light, heat, electricity, and life.

105. We will teach to our disciples in the this course of Kundalini Yoga all of the secret science of Maha-Kundalini so that they can awaken all of their occult powers and convert themselves into Logoi, into Dhyan-Choans, into Buddhas of Christic nature.

106. While the couple is in sexual copulation, the woman as well as the man should chant the pranava **Kandil, Bandil, R**.

107. The male should be seated at the right of the female.

108. While seated, male and female should chant this sacred pranava of Maha-Kundalini.

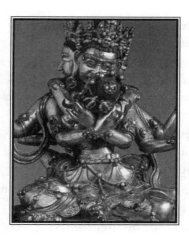

109. The seven planetary Logoi officiated the rituals of Maha-Kundalini in their temples in the dawn of the Mahamanvantara.

110. I, Samael Aun Weor, was a witness of the dawn of the Mahamanvantara.

111. I still remember when I was visiting the sacred temples of the Chaos.

112. An ineffable lady was next to a Logos in every temple.

113. Indeed, the separated sexes did not exist; however, the ineffable gods knew how to polarize themselves in accordance with the necessities of the moment.

114. The Elohim or Prajapatis are hermaphrodites.

115. One Prajapati or Elohim can draw forth his masculine or feminine polarity; they know how to polarize themselves.

116. This is how the seven planetary Logoi could draw forth their masculine aspect.

117. This is how their Isis could draw forth their feminine aspect.

118. Now our disciples will understand how inside each one of the temples of the Chaos the gods worked in couples, chanting the rhythms of fire.

119. Groups of children (Prajapatis or Elohim) formed choruses with these ineffable couples.

120. The sacred fire emerges from the brain of the Father and from the bosom of the Mother.

121. This coenobium of the sacred fire fecundated Mulaprakriti so that life could emerge.

122. The raw matter of the Great Work is the Christonic semen.

123. The raw matter of the Great Work is the mazar of the gods, the sea of milk, the fountain of milk and of the coagulations, the water of Amrita.

124. That is the sacred cow from where life emerges.

125. These are the primordial waters that are deposited within our sexual glands.

126. The Verb of the gods fecundated the chaotic matter so that life could emerge.

127. The throat is a uterus where the Word is gestated.

128. The throat is the sexual organ of the gods.

129. The sexual magic of the Word fecundated the chaotic matter so that life could emerge.

130. The creation of the universe was the outcome of the sexual magic of the Word.

131. The universe was elaborated with the type of Anu atom within the profound bosom of Parabrahman.

132. The Anu atom cannot be multiplied or divided in the pro-genital or primogenital state.

133. All the atoms of the universe are nothing but passing vestures of the primordial Anu atom.

134. This primordial Anu atom is Nirvanic.

135. The objective material universe is born from a Nirvanic condensation.

136. The entire universe is granulated Fohat.

137. The entire material universe is elaborated with the granulations of Fohat.

Chapter 2

The Degrees of Power of the Fire

1. The cerebrospinal nervous system is formed by: cerebrum, cerebellum, medulla oblongata, and spinal medulla.

2. The medulla oblongata connects the cerebellum with the sacred spinal medulla.

3. The medulla oblongata is intimately related with all of the so-called "involuntary functions" of our organic system.

4. The medulla begins on the top of the spinal canal and ends in the first vertebra of the coccygeal region.

5. The spinal medulla is a cord of gray and white material.

6. The gray matter is in the center of the spinal

medulla and the white matter in its periphery.

7. The gray matter is formed in its conjunction by innumerable nervous cells and a multitude of nervous fibers.

8. The white matter is formed by nervous medullar matter.

9. All of this matter looks as if it is suspended from the medullar canal.

10. The nourishment of this fine medullar matter is performed by means of the delicate web of membranes that are around it.

11. The medulla and the brain are surrounded by a powerful liquid mentioned by Mr. Leadbeater in one of his books.

12. This marvelous fluid protects the medulla and the brain.

13. The medulla is totally protected by a marvelous covering of innumerable tissues of greasy matter.

14. The medulla is divided into two symmetrical parts, which are completely demarcated by two

caesuras: the caesura of Silvio and the caesura of Rolando.

15. The "canalis centralis" exists throughout the length of the medulla.

16. The Brahmanadi runs throughout the length of this medullar canal from the chakra Muladhara until the chakra Sahasrara.

17. The Kundalini rises throughout this nadi until the Brahmarandhra.

18. The Brahmarandhra is septuple in its internal constitution.

19. Each one of our seven bodies has its own spinal medulla and its Brahmanadi.

20. The Kundalini is constituted by seven serpents.

21. These seven serpents are the seven radicals.

22. These seven serpents of Devi Kundalini are the seven brethren of Fohat. These

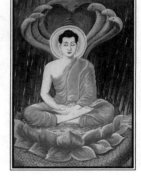

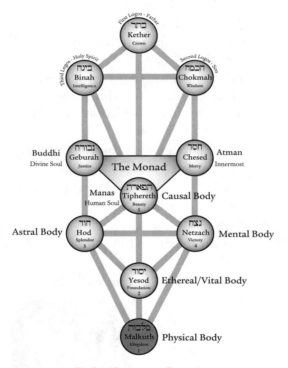

THE SEVEN BODIES ON THE TREE OF LIFE

seven serpents of Devi Kundalini are
the seven degrees of power of the fire.

23. The septenary constitution of the
human being is:

1. Atman: the Innermost

2. Buddhi: the consciousness, the
Divine Soul

3. Superior Manas: the Human
Soul, Willpower, Causal body

4. Inferior Manas: the mind, Mental
body

5. Kama-Rupa: the body of desires,
the Astral body

6. Linga-sarira: the Vital (Ethereal)
body

7. Sthula-sarira: the physical body

24. Each one of these seven bodies has its
own spinal medulla, its Shushumna-
nadi, and its Brahmanadi.

25. Seven are the serpents: two groups
of three with the coronation of the
seventh tongue of fire that unites us
with the One, with the Law, with the
Father.

26. These are the seven levels of
knowledge.

27. These are the seven doorways of the seven great Initiations of Major Mysteries.

28. Only the terror of love and law reign throughout these seven doorways.

29. The human being raises the first serpent through the first Initiation of Major Mysteries.

30. The human being raises the second serpent through the second Initiation of Major Mysteries, and likewise successively.

31. The human being who raises the seventh serpent converts himself into a Maha-Chohan.

32. The spinal medulla penetrates the fourth ventricle of the brain, and after having passed through the third and fifth ventricle, reaches the chakra Sahasrara, which is situated in the superior part of the crown of the head.

33. The vertebral column has 33 vertebrae.

34. The cervical region is formed by seven vertebrae, the dorsal by twelve, the

lumbar by five, the sacrum by five, and the coccygeal by four vertebrae.

35. These vertebrae are connected among themselves by fibro-cartilaginous cushions.

36. These vertebrae are septuple in their constitution, because they are in each one of the seven bodies of the human being.

37. Each one of these vertebrae corresponds, in the internal worlds, to a holy chamber.

38. As the human being causes the Kundalini to rise throughout his spinal medulla, he is penetrating into each one of the holy chambers of the temple.

39. Each one of these 33 chambers is septuple in its internal constitution.

40. The seven aspects of each one of these 33 holy chambers exactly correspond to the seven degrees of power of the fire.

41. We are penetrating within the first aspect of each one of these 33 holy chambers with the first degree of power of the fire.

42. We penetrate within the second aspect of each one of these 33 holy chambers with the second degree of power of the fire, which belongs to the Ethereal body.

43. We penetrate within the 33 holy chambers of the Astral body with the third degree of power of the fire.

44. We penetrate within the 33 holy chambers of the Mental body with the fourth degree of power of the fire, and likewise successively.

45. We christify our seven bodies with the seven degrees of power of the fire.

46. We know the mysteries of the seven great Initiations of Major Mysteries with the seven degrees of power of the fire.

47. Our entire personality must be absorbed within the Purusha.

48. Our entire personality must be absorbed within the Innermost.

49. The three Thrones must be awakened to liberty and to life.

50. This is how we prepare ourselves to receive our resplendent Dragon of Wisdom, our Cosmic Chrestos, that

incessant breath from the Absolute who lives within the depth of our Being.

51. The human being is converted into a Cosmic Chrestos when he receives his resplendent Dragon of Wisdom.

52. Jesus of Nazareth converted himself into a Cosmic Chrestos when he received his resplendent Dragon of Wisdom in the Jordan.

53. John the Baptist was an initiate of the Cosmic Chrestos.

54. An eternal breath is within the heart of every life.

55. All of the breaths of life are the Great Breath emanated from the Absolute in the dawn of the Mahamanvantara.

56. All the breaths are resplendent Dragons of Wisdom.

57. The Great Breath is the Cosmic Christ, the Army of the Voice, Kwan-Yin, the Melodious Voice, Avalokiteshvara, Vishnu, Osiris, the Central Sun.

58. After having raised the seven serpents upon the staff, the human being then, after some time of work,

prepares himself to receive his resplendent Dragon of Wisdom.

59. That is the "descent of Christ into the human being."

60. I, Aun Weor*, received my resplendent Dragon of Wisdom, named Samael, Logos of the planet Mars.

61. I am the Kalkian Avatar of the new Aquarian era.

62. I am the Cosmic Christ of Aquarius.

63. I am the initiator of the new era.

64. I am Samael, the planetary genie of Mars.

* - It is necessary to understand the relationship between God, spirit, soul, and body. Samael Aun Weor is the bodhisattva (awakened soul) of Samael, a controversial angel in Kabbalah. Samael Aun Weor is the name of the human soul (Tiphereth; Psykhe, Manas, or the Bodhisattva), who is not the same entity as the Innermost (Chesed, the Inner Buddha, Pneuma, Atman, Abraham), or what is commonly called "God," our "Father who is in secret" (Kether, the Logos, Brahma, Dharmakaya). Samael Aun Weor repeated many times that he, the terrestrial person, was no one important, but his Inner Being is the archangel known by many names, such as Samael, Ares, Mars, etc., the Logos of the strength of Mars, that aspect of divinity that wages war against impurity and injustice. This angel is described in the book of Revelation. You can learn more about this at SamaelAunWeor.info

Chapter 3
The Two Witnesses

1. *"And the angel that talked with me came again, and waked me, as a man that is wakened out of his sleep.*

2. *"And said unto me, What seest thou? And I said, I have looked, and behold a candlestick all of gold, with a bowl upon the top of it, and his seven lamps thereon, and seven pipes to the seven lamps, which are upon the top thereof:*

3. *"And two olive trees by it, one upon the right side of the bowl, and the other upon the left side thereof."* - Zechariah 4:1-3

4. *"Then answered I, and said unto him, What are these two olive trees upon the right side of the candlestick and upon the left side thereof?*

5. *"And I answered again, and said unto him, What be these two olive branches which through the two golden pipes empty the golden oil out of themselves?*

6. *"And he answered me and said, Knowest thou not what these be? And I said, No, my lord.*

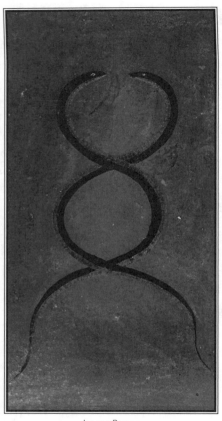

IDA AND PINGALA

7. *"Then said he, These are the two anointed ones, that stand by the Lord of the whole earth."* - Zechariah 4:11-14

8. The two olive branches that through the two golden pipes empty the golden oil out of themselves are the two nadis Ida and Pingala.

9. In the male, Ida rises from the right testicle and Pingala from the left testicle.

10. In the female, Ida and Pingala rises from the ovaries.

11. These (Ida and Pingala) are the two olive trees (of the temple), the two candlesticks standing before the God of the earth. These are the two witnesses, *"and if any man will hurt them, fire proceedeth out of their mouth and devoureth their enemies."* - Revelation 11:4, 5

12. The solar and lunar atoms of our seminal energy rise through these two ganglionic cords named Ida and Pingala.

13. The right nasal cavity is related with Pingala. The left nasal cavity is related with Ida.

14. It is stated that the solar atoms penetrate through the right nasal cavity and that the lunar atoms penetrate through the left nasal cavity.

15. The yogis and yoginis who have not been initiated in the school of internal mysteries practice Pranayama with the intention of attracting into the magnetic field of their nose millions of solar and lunar atoms from the exterior world.

16. However, the yogi/yogini-esotericist-initiate does not search outside in the world of Maya. The yogi/yogini-esotericist-initiate searches within their Self.

17. When a yogi/yogini-esotericist-initiate practices Pranayama, they only want to make their sexual energy rise from their testicles/ovaries to the sacred chalice of their brain.

18. Pranayama is an esoteric system in order to transmute the semen into Christic energy.

19. Pranayama is a system of transmutation for the sexual energy.

20. When the yogi/yogini-esotericist-initiate inhales the Prana or Vital Christ through the right nasal cavity and exhales the Prana through the left nasal cavity, and vice versa, when he inhales through the left nasal cavity and exhales through the right nasal cavity, what he wants is not to attract external atoms as the profane believe, but rather, to raise the solar and lunar atoms from his testicles to the magnetic field at the root of his nose.

21. The clairvoyant who observes the ganglionic cords Ida and Pingala of a yogi/yogini in the moments of practicing Pranayama will see the pure waters of Amrita, the primordial waters of Genesis, ascending through these two nadis.

22. Swara is the breathing science. Swara is the sacred science of respiration.

23. The mantras for the inhalation are **TON-SAH-HAM** and the mantras for the exhalation are **TON-RA-HAM**, whose hind-ends (in the testes and ovaries) correspond to the rhythmic contraction and expansion

of the undifferentiated cosmic matter, Prakriti, Mulaprakriti. (See *Biorhythm* by the Master Huiracocha).

24. Thus, from the mantra **SVA-RA** is formed the sublime Swara of which is stated in the fifteenth verse of the Sivagama: "The Vedas and the Shastras (sacred books of Hinduism) are within the Swara. The three worlds are within the Swara. Swara is the reflection of Parabrahman (the Unique Whole, the Absolute). This is why some authors state: Swara is life. And they add, Swara is music..." (*Biorhythm* by the Master Huiracocha, Dr. Arnold Krumm-Heller, page 72).

25. Swara afterwards forms the base of the Tattvas, since these are the five modifications of the Great Breath. (*Biorhythm*).

26. Now and then, the Great Breath is the Cosmic Christ, Avalokiteshvara, Kwan-Yin, the Melodious Voice, the Army of the Voice, whose head is a Paramarthasatya known in this humanity with the name of Jesus Christ.

27. Jesus Christ is the greatest initiate who has come into the world.

28. The Army of the Voice is the "Merkabah." The coachman of that chariot is Jesus Christ, the divine Rabbi of Galilee.

29. Jesus Christ is an inhabitant of the Absolute who renounced the happiness of SAT, the Unmanifested, to come into the world with Swara, the reflection of Parabrahman.

30. Therefore, Pranayama is the Christic science of the Great Breath or Cosmic Chrestos.

31. That great universal Breath of Life, the Cosmic Christ, abides within our Christonic semen.

32. The yogi/yogini works with the Great Breath or Cosmic Chrestos that is deposited within the Christonic semen when they are practicing Pranayama.

33. Pranayama (a practice that consists of making profound inhalations of air, and retaining the inhaled air as much as possible, and afterwards exhaling the air until emptying the lungs), also

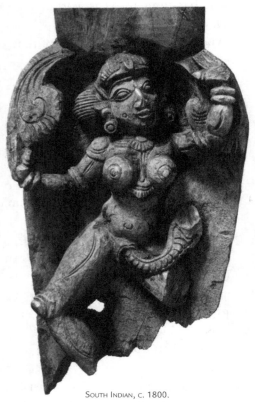

SOUTH INDIAN, C. 1800.

"Kundalini is absolutely sexual."

teaches about the poles of the energy: one masculine pole located in the brain (cerebrospinal nervous system) and the feminine pole in the heart (grand sympathetic nervous system). Thus, as when we form two poles in the space through a magneto, we create new energies and these forcedly are giving birth to a third pole; likewise, we affirm that the third pole is Devi Kundalini, which, from the union of the solar and lunar atoms, is born within the Triveni, situated in the coccyx.

34. These two polarities, masculine and feminine—from the Great Breath— prove the sexuality of Prana and Kundalini.

35. Kundalini is absolutely sexual.

36. People have the tendency of seeing sex as something filthy and horribly passionate. The yogi/yogini is ahead of Dsa, Usthi, Uste (desire) and reverently prostrates before the Gnostic mysteries of sex, because they consider that sex is a sacred function of Devi Kundalini.

37. The yogi/yogini knows that the waters of Amrita (Christonic semen) are the habitat of fire.

38. The yogi/yogini knows that the entire force of the Solar Logos abides within the seed of any plant, animal and human.

39. The yogi/yogini knows that sex is a holy force and that it must not be corrupted with fornication.

40. The respiration through the right nasal cavity is called Suria or Pingala. We cause through this respiration the ascension of the solar atoms from our seminal system.

41. The respiration through the left nasal cavity is called Chandra or Ida. We cause through this respiration the ascension of the lunar atoms from our seminal system.

42. We reinforce the Three Breaths of pure Akasha with the exercises of Pranayama. These Three Breaths are combined with the solar and lunar atoms of our seminal system to awaken Devi Kundalini.

43. Prana is the Vital Christ or Great Breath. That Vital Christ is modified into Akasha, within which the Son, the First Begotten, the Purusha of every human being, is hidden.

44. Akasha is modified into Ether, and the Ether is transformed into Tattvas. The Tattvas are the origin of fire, air, water, and earth.

45. Therefore, everything that exists, everything that has been, and everything that shall be comes from the Great Breath, the Cosmic Christ, the Army of the Voice, whose supreme commander is Jesus Christ.

46. Paranishpanna (absolute happiness) without Paramartha (awakened consciousness) is not happiness.

47. Jesus Christ attained Paramartha and Paranishpanna; nonetheless, he renounced the happiness of the Unmanifested Absolute to come and save human beings and gods.

48. When the Elohim or glorious Dhyanis started to weave in the loom of God, they cried with pain when contemplating the twilight of the

Uncreated Light that seemed to sink as a frightful setting sun.

49. Then Jesus Christ, the great Paramarthasatya, passed through the Dhyani-pasa and came into the cosmic garden to save the gods, whose innumerable virginal sparks or Jivas are devolving and evolving during this Mahakalpa.

50. I, Samael Aun Weor, was a witness of all of these things. I saw when that Great Being entered the sanctuary and signed a pact of salvation for human beings and he crucified himself on his cross.

51. I witnessed the dawn of the Mahamanvantara and give testimony of all of these things.

52. Later on, at the dawn of the fourth round, the Master sent his Buddha in order for him to prepare himself in this valley of tears. That Buddha is his soul called Jesus.

53. And his Buddha lit his seven eternal lamps.

54. And his Buddha raised his seven serpents throughout the seven canals of the candlestick.

55. Thus, when his Buddha Jesus of Nazareth was prepared there in the Jordan, his resplendent Dragon of Wisdom entered within him in order to preach to human beings and gods.

56. The sacrifice already happened on that occasion. The commander of all Cosmic Christs, Jesus of Nazareth, already washed with his blood all the sins of the sanctuary and signed the pact between human beings and Kwan-Yin, the Army of the Voice, Vishnu, Osiris, the Great Breath.

57. Jesus is the supreme conciliator between the human being and Divinity.

58. The Nadis Ida and Pingala are the subtle conductors of Shushumna-Prana, the Christic sexual energy.

59. Ida and Pingala join the nadi Shushumna in the chakra Muladhara.

60. The union of these three nadis in the chakra Muladhara is named Mukta

Triveni. This encounter of nadis is repeated in the chakra Anahata and Ajna.

61. Ida is cold and Pingala is hot.

62. The nadi Pingala is intimately related with the functions of organic assimilation.

63. Ida is of a pale color and Pingala of a red igneous color.

64. The yogi/yogini can retain the Prana that circulates through the nadi Shushumna at the point called Brahmarandhra, located in the frontal fontanel of newborn babies.

65. Thus, this is how the yogi/yogini can defy death and live entire ages.

66. However, this is only possible for the yogi/yogini that has received the Elixir of Long Life.

67. That elixir is a gas and a liquid.

68. That white-colored gas is electropositive and electronegative.

69. That gas remains deposited in the vital depth; thus the initiate can keep his physical body alive for millions of years.

70. This liquid makes the physical body subtle.

71. Thus, the physical body is absorbed within the Ethereal body and becomes indestructible.

72. The nadis Ida and Pingala are found side to side of the spinal medulla.

73. These nadis entwine around the spinal medulla in similar shape to the number eight.

74. The heavenly path is inside the nadi Shushumna.

75. The Kundalini ascends throughout the Brahmanadi.

76. The Brahmanadi is found situated inside another very subtle canal that runs throughout the length of the spinal medulla and is known with the name of Chitra.

77. The seven chakras known with the names of Muladhara, Svadhisthana, Manipura, Anahata, Vishuddha, Ajna, and Sahasrara are over this nadi Chitra.

78. Buddhi (the Divine Soul) becomes united with Shiva (the Innermost) when the Kundalini reaches the

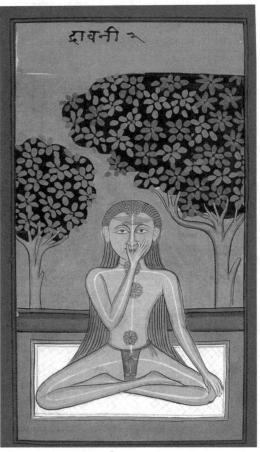

PRANAYAMA

chakra Sahasrara. This is the First Initiation of Major Mysteries.

Exercise of Pranayama

79. Let the disciple sit down on the ground, crossing his legs in the oriental style. This position is called Padmasana in India.

80. Shut the left nasal cavity with the index finger and inhale the Prana through the right nasal cavity.

81. Now, retain the air while shutting both nasal cavities with the index finger and the thumb.

82. Exhale the air through the left nasal cavity while shutting the right nasal cavity; inhale now through the left nasal cavity. Retain the air again and exhale through the right nasal cavity.

83. When you are inhaling the air, imagine the sexual energy ascending through the nadi related with the nasal cavity through which you are inhaling the Prana.

84. Think of the Three Breaths of pure Akash descending through the nadis Shushumna, Ida, and Pingala when you are sending the inhaled Prana

downwards, so to awake the chakra Muladhara where the Kundalini abides.

85. Prana is the purifying fire that cleans the scoria which plugs the nadis.

86. The veils of Rajas and Tamas are dissipated with the sexual transmutation in Pranayama.

87. The mind of the student is prepared for Dharana, Dhyana, and Samadhi with the practice of Pranayama.

88. The disciple should practice Pranayama ten minutes daily.

89. The disciple should drink a glass of milk or eat any light food after he finishes the practice.

90. The disciples can also practice while standing firm on their feet.

91. The disciple should slowly inhale and exhale with his mind very well concentrated in his practice of Pranayama.

92. There are many Asanas and exercises of Pranayama, but the former exercise of Pranayama is enough for the transmutation of the student's sexual energies.

93. The disciples can also sit on a comfortable sofa to perform his practices.

94. Before starting his practices, the disciple must pray to his Innermost by meditating profoundly on Him.

95. The disciple must be profoundly concentrated in his chakra Muladhara and begging to his Purusha (the Innermost) for the awakening of the Kundalini.

96. The oriental Yoga gives a great variety of exercises for Pranayama.

97. Let us see: deep breathing exercise, Sukha Purvaka (easy, comfortable) Pranayama during walking, Pranayama during meditation, Rhythmical breathing, Suryabheda, Ujjayi, Sitkari, Sitali, Bhastrika, Bhramari, Murchha, Plavini, Kevala Kumbhaka, etc.

98. All of these innumerable varieties of practices and Asanas (postures) served for the descending arch of the evolving life; yet, now we are starting an ascending arch of evolution, and therefore, that enormous quantity of

postures and exercises are antiquated for the new Aquarian era.

99. Now the yogi/yogini of the new Aquarian era live a life of intense activity within the cities, and they do not need to withdraw into the solitary forests, because we are initiating the new Aquarian era. This era is of sociability, cooperation, and confraternity amongst all human beings without distinction of schools, races, sexes, castes, or religions.

100. All the exercises of Pranayama can be executed in our own home without too many complications, and without abandoning the execution of all the responsibilities with our family, society, and humanity.

101. The yogi/yogini must be absolutely chaste, otherwise they will fail totally.

Chapter 4
The Yogic Matrimony

1. In our former chapter we studied the esotericism of Pranayama and we realized that it is a scientific system of transmutation for celibate people (singles).

2. The Swara (breathing science) is totally sexual.

3. The breathing science is reinforced by the sexual union of the spouses.

4. There is an act of sexual magic by means of which we can totally awaken and develop Devi Kundalini.

5. The formula is the following: introduce the virile member into the feminine vagina and withdraw from the sexual act without spilling the semen (without reaching the orgasm).

6. The refrained desire will transform the semen into light and fire.

7. The seminal vapors open the inferior orifice of the spinal medulla which in common and ordinary people is found completely closed.

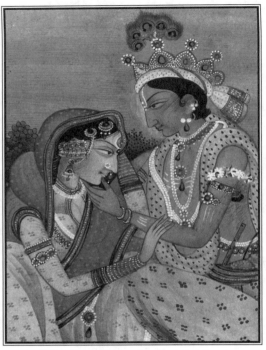

KRISHNA (THE HINDU CHRIST) AND HIS BELOVED RADHA

"This is the secret of the Vedas."

8. This labor is developed under the direction of certain Devas who govern the elemental department of the cedars of the forest.

9. Devi Kundalini enters through the orifice of the nadi Shushumna.

10. Pranayama is totally reinforced with the practices of sexual magic.

11. The Great Breath is totally sexual.

12. Sexual Magic reinforces the Great Breath within us.

13. This is how Devi Kundalini evolves, develops and progresses until attaining the union with the Lord Shiva.

14. Gautama Buddha practiced his cult of sexual magic with his beautiful spouse Yasodhara.

15. Only the one who has drank the juice of the plant of the moon (soma) can be a Brahmin.

16. This plant of the moon is sex, whose juice (soma) awakens the Kundalini in us.

17. This is the secret of the Vedas.

18. The Master Helena Petrovna Blavatsky was a great yogini.

19. This great Master, after having widowed, had to get married again in the last years of her life in order to attain her total realization and the development of all of her powers.

20. A certain disciple once asked the Master Morya, "Master, you already arose the seven serpents upon the staff; then why do you have a spouse?

    The Master answered, "Because I got her before awakening my fires, and I need her to enliven my fires."

21. The refrained desire makes our sexual energies rise through Ida and Pingala; thus, finally, the lunar and solar atoms from Ida and Pingala join in the triveni to awaken Devi Kundalini.

22. During the amorous caresses, the electricity and universal fire of life are accumulated in our atmosphere.

23. If human beings ejaculate their semen, then, as electric batteries, they discharge themselves and totally fail in the Great Work of the Father.

24. The refrained desire causes the transmutation of the seminal liquor

into Christic energy that raises
through the nadis Ida and Pingala.

25. The yogi/yogini withdraws from their
spouse before the spasm or orgasm to
avoid the seminal ejaculation.

26. The seminal fire ascends through
the nadi Shushumna throughout the
length of the Brahmanadi.

27. This is how the esotericist-yogi/yogini
realizes their Self totally, in depth,
as Masters of the Cosmic Day, as
Masters of the Mahamanvantara.

28. The yogi/yogini of the new Aquarian
era realize their Self through the
sexual act.

29. The times in which yogis needed to
withdraw into the jungle to practice
their esoteric exercises are gone.

30. Now yogis realize their Self though
the sexual act.

31. The motto of the new Aquarian era is
human cooperation.

32. Yogis must live within society, serving
their brothers and sisters and living
with happiness and optimism.

33. The new Aquarian era does not admit
hermit-yogis.

34. The Age of Maitreya is the age of association and confraternity among all human beings.

35. Sex is terrifically divine, and therefore the yogi/yogini must clean their mind from all kind of desires and animal passions.

36. The person who looks at sex with repugnance defiles the terrific secret of the Vedas and the science of the Great Breath, contained in the Vedas and the Shastras.

37. The yogi/yogini who flees from the sacred mysteries of sex is still filled with desires and animal passions.

38. Angels see sex with the eyes of an angel; yet, demons see sex with the eyes of a demon, even when they dress themselves with the skin of sheep and disguise themselves as saints.

39. The yogi/yogini form their home without the necessity of violating the Sixth Commandment of the Law of God: "Thou shall not fornicate."

40. A single sperm can escape during the act of sexual magic. The [divine] lunar hierarchies can select that

sperm to fecundate the womb without the necessity of spilling the semen.

41. This is how the Lemurians engendered their children in the stony sacred patios of their temples.

42. The tenebrous ones from the [devolving] lunar path were the ones who taught human beings how to ejaculate their seminal liquor. This is how human beings sank into the darkness.

43. Now, we have to return into the sacred conception of the Holy Spirit.

44. The children of the yogi and yogini are fragments of victory, children of chastity, children engendered by Kriya-Shakti.

45. All yogis and yoginis must love their spouse and their children, and live amidst harmony, music, love, and beauty.

46. Love dignifies; love exalts the soul.

47. God shines upon the perfect couple.

48. There is nothing greater than love. Man and woman were born to love each other.

49. The true yogi and yogini convert their home into an Eden of ineffable joys.

50. The divine priestess is the woman of the yogi, and vice versa.

51. Women convert men into ineffable gods by means of the very sweet enchantment of love, and vice versa.

52. Yogis and yoginis realize their Selves by means of love. This is better than carrying out the life of a hermit.

The Seven Chakras

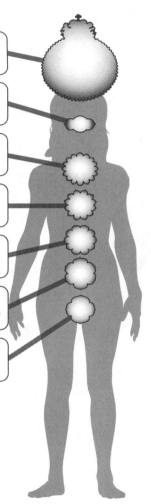

Chakra: Sahasrara
Church: Laodicea
Region: Pineal gland
Vowel: I (ee)

Chakra: Ajna
Church: Philadelphia
Region: Pituitary gland
Vowel: I (ee)

Chakra: Vishuddha
Church: Sardis
Region: Thyroid gland
Vowel: Eh

Chakra: Anahata
Church: Thyatira
Region: Heart
Vowel: O

Chakra: Manipura
Church: Pergamos
Region: Solar plexus
Vowel: U

Chakra: Svadhisthana
Church: Smyrna
Region: Prostate / Uterus
Vowel: M

Chakra: Muladhara
Church: Ephesus
Region: Sexual Organs
Vowel: S

Chapter 5
The Chakra Muladhara

1. Each one of the chakras located along the spinal medulla awakens as the Kundalini is ascending within the Nadi Chitra.

2. These seven chakras are located along the spinal medulla.

3. When the Kundalini is still enclosed within the Muladhara chakra, then these seven chakras are just hanging down.

4. However, when Devi Kundalini ascends throughout the Brahmanadi, then the marvelous petals of these chakras turn upward to Brahmarandhra, thus marvelously gleaming with the incomparable sexual fire of Kundalini.

5. Today, in this lesson, we are going to study the Muladhara chakra.

6. This chakra resides at the very base of the spinal column, and is located between the sexual organs and the anus.

7. So this chakra is located at the very root of our genital organs. It awakens in the man and in the woman when they unite their enchantment in Sexual Magic.

8. The yogi/yogini who does not have a spouse can activate the flames of his Kundalini with Pranayama and meditation. However, the complete, total, and absolute development of the seven degrees of power of the fire are only possible when practicing Sexual Magic with our priest/priestess-spouse.

9. This is why the yogini Helena Petrovna Blavatsky had to marry again in the last years of her life, long after her first husband Count Blavatsky died.

10. The seven chakras are the seven churches mentioned in the book Revelation of Saint John.

11. Now, we are studying the Muladhara chakra; this is the church of Ephesus.

12. *"Unto the angel of the church of Ephesus write: These things saith he that holdeth the seven stars in his right hand, who*

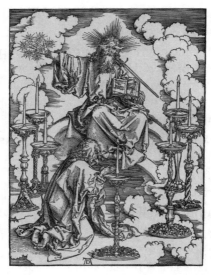

walketh in the midst of the seven golden candlesticks."

13. The one who walks in the midst of the seven golden candlesticks is our inner Christ, our inner angel.

14. The seven golden candlesticks are the seven spinal medullas, which are interrelated with our seven bodies.

15. The sacred fire ascends throughout these seven spinal medullas.

16. So, each one of our seven bodies has its own golden candlestick; that is to

say, each one has its spinal medulla
and its sacred fire.

17. We have seven serpents: two groups
of three, with the sublime coronation
of the seventh tongue of fire that
unite us with the One, with the Law,
with the Father.

18. The seven stars that our inner Christ
has in his right hand are the seven
chakras of our spinal medulla.

19. The Muladhara chakra is situated
under the Kanda, which is the exact
place where the nadis Sushumna, Ida,
and Pingala join.

20. This is the fundamental or coccygeal
chakra. This chakra nourishes all the
other chakras with its sexual energy.

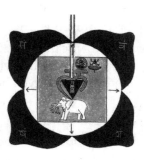

21. The Kundalini is found enclosed within the Muladhara chakra. Four nadis similar to the petals of the lotus flower emanate from this chakra.

22. The seven levels of cosmic consciousness are situated underneath the church of Ephesus.

23. The mantra of this chakra is **Bhur**.

24. The mantras **Dis**, **Das**, **Dos** must be vocalized by prolonging the sound of the vowels and letter **S**.

25. **Dis**, **Das**, **Dos** are the mantras that— when vocalized in sexual magic— awaken the Kundalini.

26. *"I know thy works, and thy labor, and thy patience, and how thou canst not bear them which are evil; and thou hast tried them which say they are Apostles, and are not, and hast found them liars."* - Revelation 2:2

27. The root of good and evil is found in the church of Ephesus.

28. There are many who say they are Apostles and are not, because they are fornicators.

29. *"Remember, therefore, from whence thou art fallen, and repent, and do the first*

works; or else I will come unto thee quickly and will remove thy candlestick out of it's place, except thou repent and sadness will afflict thy heart." - Revelation 2:5

30. When the human being ejaculates his semen (reaches the orgasm), the Kundalini then descends one or more vertebrae in accordance with the magnitude of the fault.

31. Thus, *"I will remove thy candlestick out of his place, except thou repent."*

32. To re-conquer the power of the vertebrae lost in one ejaculation is very hard and difficult.

33. This is why our Lord the Christ told me: "The disciple must not let himself fall, because the disciple who lets himself fall has to struggle very hard to recover what he has lost."

34. *"He that hath an ear, let him hear what the Spirit saith unto the churches: To him that overcometh will I give to eat of the Tree of Life which is in the midst of the Paradise of God."* - Revelation 2:7

35. There are two trees: the Tree of the Science of Good and Evil, and the Tree of Life.

36. The Tree of the Science of Good and Evil is the sexual force.

37. The Tree of Life is the inner Christ of each human being.

38. The Tree of the Science of Good and Evil must be transformed into the Immolated Lamb of the Heavenly Jerusalem.

39. This is only possible when we inebriate ourselves with the aroma of that forbidden fruit that is pleasant to the sight and of a delectable aspect, of which God said: *"Thou shalt not eat of it: for in the day that thou eatest thereof thou shalt surely die."*

40. We must always withdraw from our spouse before the orgasm; thus, we avoid the seminal ejaculation. This is how the chakra Muladhara awakens. This is how Devi Kundalini awakens.

41. This is how we transform the Tree of Science of Good and Evil into the Immolated Lamb.

42. This is how we transform into living Christs, and we eat of the Tree of Life that is in the midst of the paradise of our God.

43. The Muladhara chakra is related with the Tattva Prithvi. Whosoever totally awakens this chakra and attains in-depth realization can receive the Elixir of Long Life and preserve the physical body for millions of years.

44. The Kundalini grants us knowledge of the past, present, and future.

45. In India, there is an evil order of Kula of the tenebrous goddess Kali. This is an order of black magic.

46. These dismal yogis/yoginis fornicate; they ejaculate their semen; they violate the Sixth Commandment of the law of God. This is how they negatively awaken their Kundalini.

47. When the yogi/yogini ejaculates their semen, then the Kundalini descends one or more vertebrae in accordance with the magnitude of their fault.

48. The black magicians ejaculate their semen during their practices of negative Sexual Magic.

49. Millions of solar atoms are lost in the ejaculation of the seminal fluid. These Solar atoms are replaced by billions of satanic atoms collected

from the inner atomic infernos of the human being. These satanic atoms are collected by means of the peristaltic spasmic movements of the sexual organs after fornication (after the orgasm).

50. The satanic atoms intend to ascend through the Brahmanic cord; however, the three Akashic breaths precipitate them downward to the coccyx towards the Muladhara chakra.

51. Then a certain atom in the Muladhara chakra enters into activity. Thus the Kundalini, instead of going upward throughout the Brahmanadi, goes downward to the atomic infernos of the human being and forms in the Astral body the tail (the Kundabuffer Organ) with which Satan is represented.

52. During the act of Sexual Magic, the three pure Akashic breaths are reinforced by the human will; thus, they can be for us a blessing or a curse.

53. If the yogi/yogini ejaculates their semen, then they will convert

themselves into tenebrous tantric personalities of the lunar path.

54. Those tantric personalities are totally separated from their Purusha; that is to say, they are totally separated from their Innermost or Jivatma.

55. Every personality who is separated from their Innermost sinks themselves into the lunar abysses, and little by little they disintegrate within the most terrible desperation. This is the Second Death cited in the book Revelation of Saint John.

56. But when the yogi/yogini withdraws from their spouse before the spasm, then the solar and lunar atoms multiply themselves and ascend through the nadis Ida and Pingala upward to the chalice (the encephalon).

57. Finally, the solar and lunar atoms meet in the coccyx; then the three pure Akashic breaths that descend throughout the sacred rod (spine) of the yogi/yogini awaken Devi Kundalini, so that they may raise her throughout the Brahmanadi.

58. The bamboo reed symbolizes our spinal column.

59. Thus this is how the moment in which Devi Kundalini and the Lord Shiva become united arrives in order to transform us into Masters of High Mysteries of the great White Universal Brotherhood.

60. Thus the woman* (Maya-Shakti) is the door into Eden; let us love her! Blessed be the woman (Maya-Shakti)!

* Editor's note: Shorashi Puja, the adoration of the female, is to be experienced as Maya-Shakti (Cosmic Woman, Goddess).

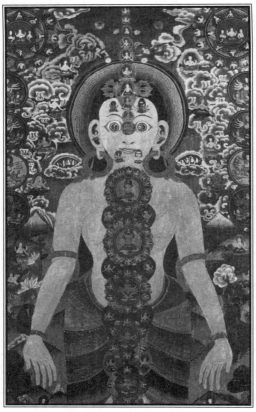

"This is how the Sadhaka penetrates all the states
of cosmic consciousness until finally acquiring
the awakening of the Absolute Consciousness."

Chapter 6
The Chakra Svadhishthana

1. The Kundalini passes through chakra after chakra.

2. This is how the different states of consciousness are opened. This is how the Sadhaka penetrates all the states of cosmic consciousness until finally acquiring the awakening of the Absolute Consciousness.

3. The yogi/yogini acquires multiple Siddhis (powers) in accordance with the awakening of his superlative consciousness.

4. In the internal worlds the word "time" is a synonym of "esoteric degrees of consciousness."

5. There are eighteen initiations: nine Initiations of Minor Mysteries and nine Initiations of Major Mysteries.

6. When in the internal worlds we state that a brother is ten years old, we are simply affirming that he is an initiate of the first Minor Mysteries.

7.   When we affirm that a disciple is ninety years old, we are asseverating that he is an initiate of the ninth initiation of Minor Mysteries.

8.   When we state that a brother is one hundred years old, we are affirming that he is in the first initiation of Major Mysteries.

9.   The ages of more than nine hundred years are Logoic ages.

10.   Experience has taught us that any Master who does not yet reached the fundamental root of the hierarchy, that is to say, that has not yet reached the ninth initiation of Major Mysteries, is very weak. That Master does not yet possess that strong and unbendable moral structure of those who already have reached Logoic ages.

11.   In order to have the right to enter into the Absolute, it is necessary to possess the age of 300,000 divine years.

12.   The last cape that a Logos wears is the Starry Mantle, with which he gains the right to enter into the Absolute.

13. Chronological time does not exist; what indeed exists is esoteric time, because life is an eternal instant.

14. All Mudras and Bandhas are totally useless for the new Aquarian era.

15. What are the Mudras useful for? It is important to transmute the sexual energies by means of love, poetry, music, and through unselfish service to this wretched suffering humanity.

16. Yet, to insert a silver tube with water into the urethra, as suggested in one of the Mudras, only destroys the sexual organs, wherein is the key to redemption.

17. A yogi/yogini can live with their physical body throughout the millions of years and move about within the pure Akasha without the necessity of cutting the inferior tendon of his tongue, as the Kechari-Mudra unfortunately teaches.

18. What is important is to attain the Elixir of Long Life and to become strong with the practice of internal meditation.

19. Gray hair and wrinkles disappear from the yogi/yogini without the necessity of performing difficult postures, such as standing on one's shoulders, raising the legs while holding the buttocks with the hands, as unfortunately is shown in the Kechari-Mudra.

20. What is important is to be pure and chaste in order to vanquish old age and death.

21. Most of all Mudras are inadequate for the new Aquarian era. It is not necessary to suffocate the Kundalini by holding the breath too much in order to awaken it; a short breath during Pranayama is enough.

22. The Kundalini awakens when we love our spouse and when following the path of the most absolute sanctity, when loving all living beings, and when we sacrifice ourselves in the Great Work of the Father.

23. What the human being needs is upright actions, upright thoughts, and upright feelings; conscientious action, conscientious word, and conscientious feeling.

24. What is important is to live life intensely in order to awaken the consciousness and to attain great realizations.

25. What is the use of standing on one's head as the Urdva-Padmasana teaches?

26. What is best is to finish with our moral defects and to sacrifice ourselves for this humanity that suffers in this "valley of tears."

27. I, Samael Aun Weor, planetary Logos of Mars, say to his Arhats: "What is best is to love, because the force of love will take us to the ineffable joy of the Absolute, where life free in its movement palpitates."

28. The Svadhishthana chakra is the abode of the Tattva Apas.

29. The elemental genie Varuna is found intimately related with this chakra.

30. The color of this chakra shines with the fire of Kundalini.

31. This chakra has six marvelous petals.

32. The mantra of this chakra is **Bhuvar**.

33. The yogi/yogini who meditates in this chakra never fears water; he learns

to command the elemental creatures of the waters and he conquers occult powers.

34. The yogi/yogini learns to recognize the different kinds of Astral entities with the awakening of this chakra.

35. The yogi/yogini conquers death with the awakening of this chakra.

36. This chakra awakens the prostatic plexus which is fundamental in the performance of practical magic.

37. An extraordinary, beautiful crescent moon is within this chakra.

38. This chakra controls the kidneys, the abdomen, and the principal organs of the lower part of the abdomen.

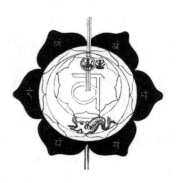

39. In the book Revelation of Saint John, this chakra is known as the church of Smyrna.

40. *"I know thy works and thy tribulations, and thy poverty, and I know the blasphemy of them which say they are Jews, and are not, but are the synagogue of Satan.*

41. *"Fear none of these things which thou shall suffer: behold, the devil shall cast some of you into prison, that ye may be tried; and ye shall have tribulation ten days; be thou faithful unto death and I will give thee a crown of life.*

42. *"He that hath an ear, let him hear what the Spirit saith unto the churches; he that overcometh shall not be hurt of the Second Death."* - Revelation 2:9-11

43. The Second Death is for the fornicators. The Tantric personalities who follow the lunar path separate themselves from their Innermost, or Purusha, and sink themselves into the sublunar spheres where they disintegrate little by little.

44. The Kula Order of the tenebrous goddess Kali came from Atlantis and passed into India. This is an order of black magic.

45. There are two types of magicians in that order: those who hate sex and those who do not, but they practice the mystical ejaculation during their negative sexual magic rites. Some of their tenebrous partisans have made this negative tantra known in the western world.

46. Those who hate the sexual force hate the Great Breath because the Great Breath is the same sexual force. The Great Breath is the Christic sexual force and those who hate this force hate the Christ. Therefore, they place themselves, in fact, on the path of black magic.

47. Our disciples are tempted and have to suffer tribulation for ten days. One has to suffer to realize the ten Sephiroth in oneself.

48. These are the ten Sephiroth of Kabbalah. Whosoever wants to self-realize the ten Sephiroth and convert their Self into a Christ has to be faithful unto death. Thus, "I will give thee a crown of life." The Inner Christ is the Incessant Eternal Breath who dwells within us.

Chapter 7
The Chakra Manipura

1. Manipura is the third chakra of our spinal medulla.

2. This chakra of our spinal medulla resides in the Nabhi Sthana (the navel area).

3. The hepatic and splenic plexuses enter into activity when this chakra awakes.

4. Ten yoga nadis emanate from this chakra.

5. The color of this chakra is like a resplendent fire.

6. The tattva Tejas is intimately related with this marvelous chakra.

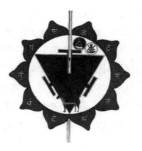

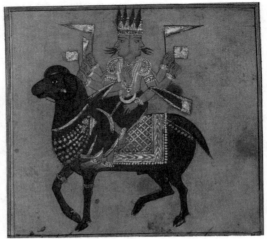

AGNI, THE GOD OF FIRE

7. The deity that rules this chakra is
   Vishnu, and the goddess Lakshmi
   is also intimately related with this
   marvelous lotus.

8. The mantra **Ram** awakens this
   marvelous chakra. The sound of each
   letter must be prolonged as follows:
   rrrrrrrrraaaaaaaammmmmmmm.

9. Our disciples could invoke the god
   Agni so that Agni can help them to
   awaken this marvelous chakra.

10. The god Agni has the appearance of a
    newborn baby and when he presents

himself dressed in formal attire,
he wears a marvelous ornamented
crystalline tunic.

11. Then we see the countenance of
this portentous being as ineffable
lightning.

12. The aura of Agni produces light and
music.

13. Agni, the god of fire, restores the
igneous powers in each one of our
seven bodies.

14. The mantra **Swa!** is pronounced as
follows:

Suuuuuuuuuaaaaaaaaaaaaaa... sua!

15. The yogi/yogini who learns to
meditate in this chakra attains the
Patala-Siddhi; they acquires great
occult powers and are free from any
type of sickness.

16. This chakra is the telepathic center or
emotional brain.

17. The mental waves of the people who
think of us reach the solar plexus;
thereafter those waves pass into our
brain.

18. Therefore, the solar plexus is our
receptor antenna.

19. Our pineal gland is our transmitter center.

20. This chakra collects the solar forces and nourishes all the other plexuses with them.

21. The yogi/yogini who awakens this chakra acquires the sense of telepathy.

22. The yogi/yogini who awakens this chakra will never fear fire and will be able to remain alive within the flames.

23. The constitution of our vertebral column is marvelous.

24. Indeed, the vertebrae are placed one above the other, forming a very beautiful pillar upon which not only our cranium is supported but all of our marvelous organism.

25. Our spinal column is a marvelous clavichord that we have to learn how to play in order to bring forth all the enchanted melodies of the Zodiac.

26. There are marvelous gaps between each pair of vertebrae, so that the spinal nerves can pass through them. These spinal nerves come from our

spinal medulla to join each one of the prodigious chakras of the grand sympathetic nervous system.

27. The yogi/yogini must keep the elasticity of the spinal column.

Practice:

28. Standing on our feet, vertical posture, with the hands placed on the waist, the yogi/yogini will turn his trunk from right to left around his waist, and thus he will keep the elasticity of the spinal column.

29. The solar plexus is the seat of Satan (inferior Astral lunar body).

30. Revelation of Saint John warns us as follows:

"I know thy works and where thou dwellest, even where Satan's seat is: and thou holdest fast my name, and hast not denied my faith, even in those days wherein Antipas was my faithful martyr, who was slain among you, where Satan dwelleth.

"But I have a few things against thee, because thou hast there them that hold the doctrine of Balaam, who taught Balac to cast a stumblingblock before the children

of Israel, to eat things sacrificed unto idols, and to commit fornication.

"So hast thou also them that hold the doctrine of the Nicolaitanes, which thing I hate. Repent; or else I will come unto thee quickly, and will fight against them with the sword of my mouth.

"He that hath an ear, let him hear what the Spirit saith unto the churches; To him that overcometh will I give to eat of the hidden manna, and will give him a white stone, and in the stone a new name written, which no man knoweth saving he that receiveth it." - Revelation 2:13 -17

31. The lunar body or inferior Astral body—called Satan in esoteric Christian language—is connected to the solar plexus.

32. Now our disciples will comprehend from where the desires of overeating and drinking alcohol come.

33. Now our brothers will understand where the craving for fornication and gluttony are born.

34. The lunar body is a remnant from our animal past.

35. The ancestral inheritance from the animal kingdom is preserved as our lower passions within the lunar body.

36. When we were animal elementals, our astral lunar (protoplasmic) body was not yet divided.

37. Yet, when we, for the first time, entered into the human kingdom, this Astral lunar body was divided in two portions, one superior, this was imbibed by the mind (inferior manas); any yogi/yogini moves consciously with this part during sleep. The other, the inferior, is called Satan in the esoteric Christian language; this is the inferior lunar Astral body (Kama-Rupa).

38. This lunar body is gigantic and deformed in perverse personalities.

39. Now our brothers and sisters will understand why our Lord the Christ said: *"Except ye be converted, and become as little children, ye shall not enter into the kingdom of heaven."* – Matthew 18:3

40. Satan is nourished with our appetites and passions. Yet, when we remove the sources of his nutrition, he becomes smaller and beautiful.

41. This is how, dear brethren, we eat of hidden manna, the bread of wisdom.

42. This is how, beloved disciples, we receive the cornerstone from the temple of the living God.

43. That cornerstone is our resplendent Dragon of Wisdom, our inner Christ; that is the Breath of the Central Sun within us.

44. This is the small white stone on which is written our holy name.

45. Repent, dear brethren, and finish with all your defects.

46. Sanctify yourselves, brethren of my Soul, so that you will not fall into the lunar abysses (Avitchi).

47. Perverse personalities are divorced from the Monad and sink themselves into the lunar abysses of the eighth sphere.

Chapter 8
The Chakra Anahata

1. This chakra has complete control over the cardiac plexus.
2. Its color is like living fire.
3. Indeed, there is a jet-black hexagonal space inside this marvelous chakra.
4. This chakra is intimately related with the Tattva Vayu.
5. The deity that rules this chakra is Isha, who controls and rules this chakra along with the Devata Kakini.
6. The Bana Linga is found intimately related with the Anahata chakra.
7. The Svayambhu Linga is intimately related with the Muladhara chakra.

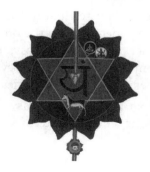

8.   The Anahata sound, or the Shabda Brahman sound, resounds within this marvelous chakra of the Nadi Sushumna.

9.   This marvelous sound is the sound of the Fohat.

10. The sound of the Fohat is the "S" which is vocalized as follows: *Sssssssssssss...* as a sweet and affable whistle.

11. The yogi/yogini who learns how to meditate in this chakra will become an absolute master of the Tattva Vayu and will be able to dissolve hurricanes and command the winds at will.

12. Some yogis state that one can float in the air and penetrate into the body of another person just by meditating on this chakra.

13. Undoubtedly, to float in the air and to penetrate into the body of another person is very easy; it can be accomplished by anybody, even if he is a beginner in these studies.

14. To float in the air is as easy as drinking a cup of water.

15. The secret is very simple; it is enough for the disciple to learn how to penetrate into the Astral plane with his physical body.

Practice

16. Disciples must slumber lightly; then very softly they must get up from their bed as if they were somnambulists; that is to say, preserving the sleepy state as a very precious treasure.

17. Thus, in this way, as the disciple walks as a somnambulist, filled with faith, they will jump with the intention of floating in the surrounding environment.

18. If the disciple achieves floating in the air, it is because their physical body have penetrated into the Astral plane. Thus, the disciple can go across space and soar to any given place of the Earth.

19. This is how we can fly with the physical body within the Astral plane.

20. While the physical body is inside the Astral plane it becomes submitted to the laws of the Astral plane but

without losing its physiological characteristics.

21. Therefore, to float in the air with the physical body can be done by anyone. What is important is to have faith, tenacity, and very much patience.

22. The cardiac fires control the spinal fires.

23. The cardiac fires control the ascent of the Kundalini.

24. The ascent of the Kundalini is performed in accordance with the merits of our heart.

25. In order to get the benefit of only one vertebra in the spinal column, the yogi must submit himself to numerous trials and terrible purifications.

26. The progress, development, and evolution of the Kundalini is very slow and difficult.

27. With only one seminal ejaculation, the Kundalini descends one or more vertebrae in accordance with the magnitude of the fault.

28. To re-conquer the powers of those vertebrae is terribly difficult.

29. The serpents of the physical and Vital bodies only reach at the level of the eyebrows, but the serpents of the Astral, Mental, Causal, Consciousness, and Atmic bodies inevitably descend from the level of the eyebrows into the heart.

30. An accessory nerve goes from the spinal medulla into the heart. Through this accessory nerve our five superior serpents pass from the frontal region of the eyebrows into the heart.

31. This fine accessory thread of our spinal medulla controls the accessory muscles of the heart and has seven holy chambers.

32. There are seven holy centers within the heart. Each one of our seven serpents is intimately related with a chamber of the heart.

33. Our disciples must have a system of purification and sanctification. The heart is the abode of our Innermost.

34. Disciples must make a list of all their defects. Then they must begin to amend them orderly and methodically.

35. The disciple could dedicate two months to amend each defect.

36. The hunter who wants to catch ten rabbits at one time will not catch a single one.

37. It is necessary to attain the most absolute sanctity and the most terrific chastity to acquire the development, progress, and evolution of the Kundalini.

38. Celibate (single) people should transmute their sexual energies with Pranayama.

39. Married people (husband and wife) do not necessarily need to practice the breathing exercises, since Pranayama is condensed for them in the practices of Sexual Magic.

40. Sexual Magic is only possible to practice between husband and wife in legitimately constituted homes.

41. Whosoever practices Sexual Magic with different persons is an adulterer and a fornicator.

42. Revelation of Saint John calls this chakra the church of Thyatira.

43. *"I know thy works, and charity, and service, and faith, and thy patience (the necessary virtues that we must have in order to open the chakra of the heart), and thy works; and the last to be more than the first.*

44. *"Notwithstanding I have a few things against thee, because thou sufferest that woman Jezebel (fornication), which calleth herself a prophetess, to teach and to seduce my servants to commit fornication, and to eat things sacrificed unto idols (theories, intellectualism, that is to say, all kinds of meal offerings offered unto idols).*

"And I gave her space to repent of her fornication; and she repented not.

"Behold, I will cast her into a bed, and them that commit adultery with her into great tribulation, except they repent of their deeds.

"And I will kill her children with death; and all the churches shall know that I am he which searcheth the kidneys and hearts: and I will give unto every one of you according to your works." - Revelation 2:19-23

45. Above the kidneys there are two plexuses that irradiate blue and white

colors in the chaste people, and a
bloody red color in the fornicators.

46. Our inner Christ searches the kidneys
and hearts and gives unto each one of
us what we deserve.

47. *"And he that overcometh, and keepeth my
works (or commandments) unto the end,
to him will I give power over the nations:*

*"Even as the power that I received of my
Father I will give him the morning star."*

- Revelation 2:26-27

Chapter 9
The Chakra Vishuddha

1. The chakra Vishuddha of our spinal medulla is situated at the base of our creative larynx.

2. This marvelous chakra is intimately related with the Tattva Akash (Ethereal element).

3. The color of this chakra is of an intense blue.

4. The laryngeal chakra belongs to the Tattva Manas.

5. The divine deity that protects this marvelous chakra is Sadashiva.

6. This marvelous chakra has sixteen beautiful petals.

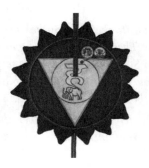

7. Indeed, the center of this chakra looks like a full moon.

8. The yogis from India affirm that by practicing meditation on this chakra, one is capable of sustaining his living physical body even during the Pralaya (cosmic night).

9. Whosoever learns to meditate on this chakra can know the highest esoteric knowledge of all the sacred books, including the Vedas.

10. The yogi/yogini who learns to meditate on this chakra will reach the grand state of Trikala Jnani—that is to say, one who is capable of knowing the past, present, and future.

11. The mantra of the Tattva Akash is **Han**. Undoubtedly, this mantra must be chanted by the yogi/yogini when meditating in this marvelous chakra.

12. *"And unto the angel of the church in Sardis write; These things saith he that hath the seven Spirits of God, and the seven stars; I know thy works, that thou hast a name that thou livest, and art dead.*

13. *"Be watchful, and strengthen the things which remain, that are ready to die: for I*

have not found thy works perfect before God.

14. *"Remember therefore how thou hast received and heard, and hold fast, and repent. If therefore thou shalt not watch, I will come on thee as a thief, and thou shalt not know what hour I will come upon thee.*

15. *"Thou hast a few names even in Sardis which have not defiled their garments; and they shall walk with me in white: for they are worthy.*

16. *"He that overcometh, the same shall be clothed in white raiment; and I will not blot out his name out of the book of life, but I will confess his name before my Father, and before his angels.*

17. *"He that hath an ear, let him hear what the Spirit saith unto the churches."* - Revelation 3:1-6

18. This chakra of the church of Sardis belongs to the sense of occult-hearing, or clairaudience.

19. The Mental Body is intimately related with the church of Sardis.

20. I, Samael Aun Weor, planetary Logos of Mars, after many Mahamanvantaras of incessant

evolution and progress, have arrived at the conclusion that the unique essential thing in life is sanctity.

21. The powers are flowers of the Soul that sprout when we have sanctified ourselves.

22. For one step that we take in the development of the chakras, we must take a thousand steps in sanctity.

23. We prepare our garden with the esoteric exercises so that we can make our marvelous chakras bloom with the perfume of sanctity.

24. The yogi/yogini must water his garden daily by finishing with all of his moral defects.

25. Each one of the petals of our lotus flowers represents certain virtues; without these virtues, the lotus flowers cannot open to receive the Sun of Truth.

26. Do not covet powers because you will sink into the lunar abysses.

27. It is better for those who do not want to sanctify themselves to withdraw from these teachings before it is too late for them.

28. The Vishuddha chakra is related with the creative word.

29. Sometimes to speak is a crime; and sometimes to be silent is also a crime.

30. There are delinquent silences and words of infamy.

31. The most difficult thing in life is to learn how to control our tongue.

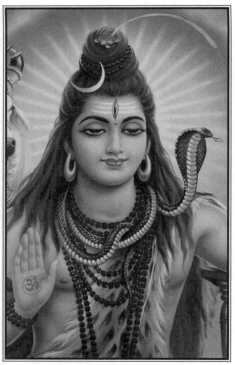

SHIVA, THE SERPENT, AND THE THIRD EYE (AJNA CHAKRA)

Chapter 10
The Chakra Ajna

1. This chakra is found connected to its marvelous center located between the eyebrows.

2. The Master who directs this center is Paramashiva.

3. The mantra that makes this chakra vibrate is **Om**: *Oooooooommmmmmmmm.*

4. This chakra has two petals.

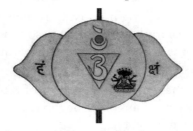

5. This marvelous chakra has a very pure white color. The cavernous plexus is the one that corresponds to this chakra.

6. The yogis from India state that one can destroy the Karmas of past lives by meditating on this chakra.

7.   I, Samael, Logos of Mars, state that nobody can mock the Law.

8.   The best that we can do is to learn how to handle our negotiations.

9.   Whosoever has capital, can pay his debts and do well in his negotiations.

10. Perform good deeds so that you may pay your debts.

11. The Lion of the Law is fought with the scale.

12. When an inferior law is transcended by a superior law, the superior law flushes away the inferior law.

13. The yogi/yogini must learn how to travel in their Astral body so that they can visit the Temple of Anubis and his 42 Judges.

14. In the temple of the Lords of Karma we can arrange our negotiations (karmic debts).

15. We can also ask for credit from the Lords of Karma, but every credit must be paid by working in the Great Work of the Father, or by suffering the unspeakable.

16. The chakra Ajna is the chakra of clairvoyance or psychic vision.

17. The plexus of this chakra is a lotus flower that sprouts from the pituitary gland. This gland is the page or light bearer of the pineal gland, where the crown of the Saints, the lotus of one thousand petals, the eye of Dangma, the eye of intuition, is situated.

18. Psychic clairvoyance by itself, without the development of the coronary chakra, could lead the yogi/yogini astray into grave errors.

19. There are billions of black magicians in the Astral and Mental planes; they disguise themselves as saints or Masters of the White Lodge to mislead the disciples or to dictate false oracles to them.

20. The only way to avoid those possible errors is by awakening intuition, whose divine diamond eye is in the lotus of a thousand petals that we are going to study in the next chapter.

21. The yogi/yogini who wants to project himself in their Astral Body must take advantage of that transition state that exists between vigil and sleep.

22. The yogi/yogini shall get up out of their bed in the very instant of falling asleep and go out of their bedroom towards the palace of the Lords of Karma to arrange their negotiations. They can go to any temple of mysteries.

23. This former procedure must be executed with actions; it is not a mere mental exercise.

24. The yogi/yogini must get up from their bed in the instants of getting slumbered, just as a somnambulist will do it.

25. Triumph is attained with patience and perseverance.

26. In former chapters, we have taught the mantras and the practices for the chakras of the spinal column.

27. However, we must not forget that the plexuses also have their mantras.

28. The powerful Egyptian mantra **Fe Uin Dagj** makes all of our plexuses vibrate. What is important is to prolong the sound of the vowels.

29. The vowels I, E, O, U, A are arranged in the following order:

I: frontal plexus

E: larynx plexus

O: cardiac plexus

U: solar plexus

A: plexus of the lungs

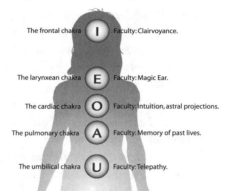

The frontal chakra — **I** — Faculty: Clairvoyance.

The larynxean chakra — **E** — Faculty: Magic Ear.

The cardiac chakra — **O** — Faculty: Intuition, astral projections.

The pulmonary chakra — **A** — Faculty: Memory of past lives.

The umbilical chakra — **U** — Faculty: Telepathy.

30. We can awaken all of our occult powers by meditating on each of these vowels, making the sound travel from between the eyebrows down to the throat, and then to the heart, the solar plexus, the legs, and finally to the feet.

31. Whosoever learns how to meditate in the Ajna chakra will acquire the eight major siddhis and the lesser thirty-two.

32.   This is the church of Philadelphia.

*"I know thy works: behold, I have set
before thee an open door, and no man can
shut it: for thou hast a little strength, and
hast kept my word, and hast not denied my
name.*

33.   *"Behold, I will make them of the synagogue
of Satan, which say they are Jews, and are
not, but do lie; behold, I will make them to
come and worship before thy feet, and to
know that I have loved thee.*

34.   *"Because thou hast kept the word of my
patience, I also will keep thee from the
hour of temptation, which shall come upon
all the world, to try them that dwell upon
the earth."* - Revelation 3:10

35.   We are tempted by billions of demons
in the Mental and Astral planes.
Many of these demons disguise
themselves as saints and masters to
tempt and deceive us.

36.   Psychic clairvoyance is set as an
open door before you; however, it is
necessary for you to acquire strength
and to keep the word of God so as to
not fall into temptation.

37. *"Because thou hast kept the word of my patience, I also will keep thee from the hour of temptation, which shall come upon the entire world, to try them that dwell upon the earth."* - Revelation 3:10

38. In the Mental Plane there are black magicians who very cunningly advise us to perform seminal ejaculation.

39. Those black magicians disguise themselves as saints and pronounce sublime speeches of love and sanctity.

40. *"Behold, I come quickly: hold that fast which thou hast, that no man take thy crown."* - Revelation 3:11

41. Those tenebrous entities advise the student to ejaculate his seminal fluid, to make his seminal liquor descend, thus taking away his crown.

42. *"Him that overcometh will I make a pillar in the temple of my God, and he shall go no more out: and I will write upon him the name of my God, and the name of the city of my God, which is new Jerusalem, which cometh down out of heaven from my God: and I will write upon him my new name.*

43. *"He that hath an ear, let him hear what the Spirit saith unto the churches."* - Revelation 3:12-13

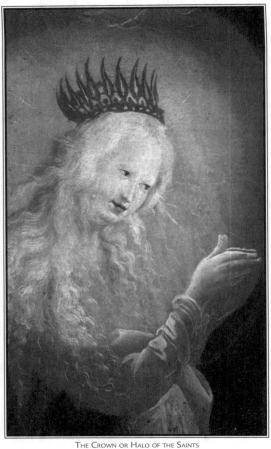

THE CROWN OR HALO OF THE SAINTS

Chapter 11

The Chakra Sahasrara

1. The chakra Sahasrara is the Crown of Saints. It is the abode of Lord Shiva and corresponds to the pineal gland.

2. The Crown of Saints is attained when Devi Kundalini reaches this chakra.

3. The Crown of Saints has twelve stars.

4. These twelve stars are twelve faculties in the true human being.

5. There are twenty-four angelic atoms in the brain; these atoms represent the twenty-four elders of the zodiac.

6. The twenty-four atomic elders of our brain ardently shine when Devi Kundalini opens the marvelous chakra.

7. This center has a thousand petals. This is the church of Laodicea.

8. The Revelation of Saint John warns us:

"I know thy works, that thou art neither cold nor hot: I would thou wert cold or hot.

So then because thou art lukewarm, and neither cold nor hot, I will spew thee out of my mouth." - Revelation 3:15-16

9. Indeed, lukewarm souls are cast out of the temple of wisdom.

10. This wisdom is for ardent souls.

11. The twenty-four atomic Elders represent the entire wisdom of the twenty-four Elders of the Zodiac.

12. The twenty-four Zodiacal Elders dressed in white garments are seated on the throne of our brain.

13. The Atom of the Father is situated in the root of our nose.

14. This is the atom of the willpower.

15. Through willpower the seven serpents of our seven bodies rise by dominating the animal impulse.

16. The Atom of the Son abides in the pituitary gland, whose exponent is the Nous Atom (the Son of Man) in the heart.

17. The atomic angel of the Holy Spirit shines within the chakra Sahasrara in the pineal gland.

18. The Atom of the Father controls the magnetic ganglionic cord of the right, Pingala.

19. The Atom of the Son governs the canal of Shushumna.

20. The Atom of the Holy Spirit governs Ida.

21. This is why the Atom of the Holy Spirit is intimately related with our sexual energies and with the rays of the Moon, which are related with human reproduction.

22. *"Behold, I stand at the door, and knock: if any man hears my voice, and opens the door, I will come in to him, and will sup with him, and he with me."* - Revelation 3:20

23. This is the wedding feast of the Lamb with the Soul.

24. When we have raised the seven serpents of fire upon the staff, He stands at the door and knocks.

25. He then comes into his temple.

26. Then He sups with us and we with Him.

27. *"To him that overcometh, will I grant to sit with me in my throne; even as I also*

*overcame and am set down with my
Father in his throne."* - Revelation: 3:21

28. This is the great event of Bethlehem;
     this is the Nativity of the heart.

29. This is the descent of Christ into the
     atomic infernos of the human being.

30. *"And there appeared a great wonder in
     heaven; a woman clothed with the sun,
     and the moon under her feet, and upon her
     head a crown of twelve stars."* - Revelation
     12:1

31. This woman dressed with the Sun is
     the Christified Soul.

32. *"And she being with child cried, travailing
     in birth, and pained to be delivered."*
     - Revelation 12: 2

33. *"And she brought forth a man child, who
     was to rule all nations with a rod of iron:
     and her child was caught up unto God, and
     to his throne."* - Revelation 12:5

34. That man-child is our inner Christ in
     gestation, that finally is born in us,
     and transforms us into Christs.

35. When Jesus received the baptism in
     the Jordan, John told him: "Jesus, you
     have received the Christ. Now you are
     a Christ."

36. There are 144,000 angelic atoms within our brain. Those angelic atoms govern all the atoms in our human organism.

37. The pituitary gland, or sixth sense, is the page, the light-bearer of the pineal gland where the Crown of the Saints is situated.

38. The internal reconcentration is more important than clairvoyance.

39. Clairvoyance is useful in all planes of consciousness.

40. Nevertheless, in the inferior planes the tenebrous entities can lead the seers astray.

41. The demons disguise themselves as angels.

42. Whosoever advises the seminal ejaculation is a black magician.

43. We open the diamond eye (the pineal gland) by means of internal reconcentration; thus, we enter into the superior worlds of fire where the truth reigns.

44. The clairvoyant who does not awaken his intuition could become a

slanderer of his neighbor and even an assassin.

45. Intuition allow us to know the internal reality of all the images that float in the Astral Light. The intuitive clairvoyant is omniscient.

46. A clairvoyant without intuition is like a ship without a compass or a ship without a steering wheel. The intuitive clairvoyant is powerful.

47. Each one of the seven chakras of the spinal column is governed by an atomic angel.

48. *"And I saw another mighty angel come down from heaven, clothed with a cloud: and a rainbow was upon his head, and his face was as it were the sun, and his feet as pillars of fire."* - Revelation 10:1

49. That mighty angel is our Innermost, crowned with a heavenly rainbow, the chakra Sahasrara of the pineal gland, whose resplendency is terribly divine.

50. *"And cried with a loud voice, as when a lion roareth: and when he had cried, seven thunders uttered their voices."* - Revelation 10:3

51. These seven thunders are the seven notes of the Lost Word that resound in the seven churches of our spinal medulla.

52. Each one of the seven angels of the seven churches sound their trumpet; they sound their key note as the sacred fire of Devi Kundalini ascends throughout the Brahmanadi of our Sushumna canal.

53. *"But in the days of the voice of the seventh angel (the atomic angel of the Sahasrara chakra) when he shall begin to sound the trumpet (which is his secret note), the mystery of God shall be consummated, as He hath declared to his servants the Prophets."* - Revelation 10:7

54. The mantra **Aum** serves to open the chakras of the grand sympathetic nervous system.

55. **Auim** for the cavernous plexus of the pituitary gland, the center of clairvoyance.

56. **Auem** for the plexus of the thyroid gland, the center of clairaudience.

57. **Auom** for the heart, the center of intuition.

58. **Aum** for the solar plexus, region of the epigastria, the telepathic center.

59. **Auam** for the chakra of the lungs that allows us to remember our past lives.

60. **Aum** is a proto-Tattvic mantra that allows us to awaken our Tattvic powers. To chant it open the mouth with the vowel A, round it with the vowel U and close it with the M.

Apply the same system for all the other mantras: **Auim**, **Auem**, **Auom**, **Aum**, **Auam**.

Chapter 12
The Seven Seals

1. When we have formed our inner Christ, He then enters into all of our vehicles through the pineal gland.

2. The inner Christ has the shape of a small child. He comes out from within his Ethereal womb to enter into our physical body through the pineal gland.

3. This is the descent of Christ into the atomic infernos of the human being.

4. This is the Nativity of the heart.

5. It is how we transform ourselves into Christs.

6. Nature does not leap; this is why our inner Christ is born within us as a small child.

7. The three wise men (the Malachim) adore him and offer him gold, incense, and myrrh.

8. These three King Magi are the Innermost, the Divine Soul, and the Human Soul (Atman-Buddhi-Manas).

9. The Star of Bethlehem is the Central Sun; it is the Great Universal Breath of Life.

10. Our inner Christ is only one particle of that spiritual Central Sun.

11. The entire universe of Pleroma, the whole thought of God, is reflected within our inner Christ.

12. Our inner Christ is the Word.

13. The Word becomes flesh within our heart with the event of Bethlehem.

14. We must clearly distinguish between the seven churches and the seven seals mentioned in Revelation.

15. The seven churches are related to the seven chakras of our spinal column.

16. The seven seals are the seven white spiritual serpents of our inner Christ.

17. These seven serpents are the spiritual part of the seven columns of fire of Devi Kundalini.

18. The seven serpents of our inner Christ are no longer fiery, but rather they are beyond fire, even though they are the cause of fire.

19. These are the seven seals of the Revelation of St. John.

20. These seven seals can be opened only by the Lamb, our inner Christ.

21. *"And I saw in the right hand of him that sat on the throne a book written within and on the backside, sealed with seven seals.*

22. *"And I saw a strong angel proclaiming with a loud voice, who is worthy to open the book, and to loose the seals thereof?*

23. *"And no man in heaven, nor in earth, neither under the earth, was able to open the book, neither to look thereon."*
- Revelation 5:1-3

24. The book is the human being, and the seven seals are the seven spiritual serpents of our Inner Christ.

25. These serpents can be raised only by the Lamb.

26. *"And I saw when the Lamb opened one of the Seals, and I heard as it were the voice of thunder, one of the four beasts saying: Come and see."* - Revelation 6:1

27. The white horse appears as the symbol of the physical body when the Lamb opens the first seal.

28. The red horse appears as the symbol of the Ethereal body when the Lamb opens the second seal.

29. The black horse appears as the symbol of the body of desires (Astral Body) when the Lamb opens the third seal.

30. The wisdom of the great Illuminati is granted to us when the Lamb opens the fourth seal. This occurs when the inner Christ takes complete possession of the Mental Body of the human being. This is the yellow horse.

31. The Human Souls appear dressed in white garments when the Lamb opens the fifth seal.

32. The sun becomes dark like black cloth and the moon becomes as blood when the Lamb opens the sixth seal. Then we are stricken with great pain, because the consciousness does not awaken but through pain and bitterness.

33. Finally, the seven atomic angels of our organism sound their trumpets in triumph, announcing victory when the Lamb opens the seventh seal.

34. *"And when he had opened the seventh seal, there was silence in heaven about the space of half an hour."* - Revelation 8:1

35. This is how the Child-God of Bethlehem grows within us.

36. The Child-God of Bethlehem has to be absorbed within all of his Bodhisattva. He performs this by raising his seven spiritual serpents.

37. So, when finally the Child-God of Bethlehem is absorbed within his Bodhisattva, he tosses his Bodhisattva back into the inner depths of the consciousness. This is how the Child-God comes from within to without, to the world of the flesh, to lean out through the five senses and to appear as a Christ among mankind, and thus to perform the Work of the Father.

38. Do not confuse the seven igneous serpents of the Soul with the seven totally Christic and spiritual serpents of the inner Christ.

39. The four horses of the Apocalypse are our four bodies of sin, the four gross bodies that constitute our inferior personality.

40. The Lamb has to raise each one of these Christic serpents in successive order; first one, then the other, and so on.

41. This work is very arduous and difficult.

42. The horseman on the white horse triumphs with his bow and arrow. Thus the physical world is dominated. The horseman on the red horse has the power to take the peace away and also to give peace because the Ethereal body is the base of the physical body.

43. The horseman on the black horse has to vanquish the weight of desire, lust, greed, and all the lower passions.

44. The name of the horseman of the yellow horse is Death; and hell and death follow him because the Mental body is constituted by the atomic infernos of the human being, where death reigns.

45. All things that exist within the human mind belong to desire; therefore, they have to die.

46. All the thought-rubbish must fall dead before the temple doorway. This is why the name of the fourth horseman is Death. And all the bitterness from hell follows him.

47. The Earth is the twin sister of Venus.

48. All the events that happen on Earth are repeated on Venus.

49. The light of the Sun reaches Earth through Venus.

50. Venus receives three times more solar light than the Earth.

51. Venus is the solar light bearer.

52. The Genie of the Earth has to receive instructions from the Genie of Venus.

53. Uriel, the Genie of Venus, is the Master of Cham-Gam, the Genie of the Earth.

54. If the light of the Sun comes to Earth through Venus, then we have no other choice than to appeal to Venus in order to be able to reach the Solar Logos.

55. Venus is Love.

56. The Kundalini develops and progresses by means of Sexual Magic.

57. God shines over the perfect couple.

58. Sexual Magic was practiced in the Eleusian mysteries, along with the holy dances and naked dances to awaken and develop Devi Kundalini.

59. In the stone courtyards of the Aztec temples, young men and women remained sexually connected, loving each other for months in order to awaken Devi Kundalini.

60. There is no greater joy than love.

61. The only way men and women can transform themselves into gods is by adoring each other. If it is not this way, it is a waste of time.

62. Venus is the first star that shines before the sunrise.

63. Venus is the first star that shines when the sun sets.

64. Venus is the Light-bearer.

65. Venus is love.

66. God shines over the beings who love each other.

Chapter 13
Internal Meditation

1. Internal meditation is a scientific system to receive information.

2. When the wise submerges into meditation, he searches for information.

3. Meditation is the daily bread of the wise.

4. Meditation has different steps.

    a. Asana (posture of the body)

    b. Pratyahara (serene mind)

    c. Dharana (internal concentration)

    d. Dhyana (internal meditation)

    e. Samadhi (ecstasy)

5. Firstly, we must place our body in a very comfortable position.

6. We have to place our mind in serenity before starting our concentration; that is to say, we have to remove every type of thought from our mind.

7. After having accomplished the former steps, we then rise up to the steps of Dharana, Dhyana, and Samadhi.

8.   Whosoever follows the path of Jnana Yoga converts himself into a Sannyasin of thought.

9.   First, we concentrate our mind in the physical body; then after meditating profoundly about the nature of this marvelous vehicle, we discard it from the mind by saying, "I am not the physical body."

10. Then, we concentrate our thought on our Ethereal body, and we discard it by saying, "I am not the Ethereal body."

11. Then after, we meditate in the Astral and Mental bodies.

12. The Astral and Mental bodies are the two columns of the temple that rest upon the cubic stone of Yesod. That cubic stone is the Ethereal body. The disciple has to pass between those two columns of the temple.

13. Those two columns are Jachin and Boaz—one black and the other white.

14. The word INRI is written with characters of fire upon those columns.

15. This word INRI is a password that allows us to pass between the two columns of the temple to function within the World of the Mist of Fire without material vehicles of any type.

16. The disciple will meditate profoundly on these two columns, which are the Astral and Mental bodies. The disciple will slumber profoundly while mentally chanting the mantra INRI, prolonging the sound of each letter by imitating the sharp sound of the crickets of the forest, thus, until achieving that sound, until giving unto the letters that sharp sound, a sound synthesis like a prolonged "S," as follows:

Sssssssssssssssssssssssssssssss......

17. It is necessary to identify oneself with that sibilant very sharp sound, similar to the most elevated note that a fine flute can give.

18. The cricket was considered sacred and was sold in golden cages at very high prices in the august Rome of the Caesars.

19. If we can have that little creature close to our ears and meditate

profoundly in its sound, then the sharp note that the cricket emits would awake in our brain the same sound.

20. Then we could rise from our bed with our Astral body and travel towards the Gnostic Church with complete consciousness.

21. That is the subtle voice mentioned by Apollonius of Tyana. That is the still small voice that Elijah heard in the entrance in of the cave.

22. Let us read some verses of the Bible:

"And he said, Go forth, and stand upon the mount before the LORD. And, behold, the LORD passed by, and a great and strong wind rent the mountains, and brake in pieces the rocks before the LORD; but the LORD was not in the wind: and after the wind an earthquake; but the LORD was not in the earthquake:

23. *"And after the earthquake a fire; but the LORD was not in the fire: and after the fire a still small voice.*

24. *"And it was so, when Elijah heard it that he wrapped his face in his mantle, and went out, and stood in the entrance of the cave.*

And, behold, there came a voice unto him, and said, What doest thou here, Elijah?"
- 1 Kings 29:11-13

25. The slumbering disciple will meditate profoundly on the black column (the Astral body) and will try to hear the still, small voice, while saying, "I am not the Astral body."

26. The disciple will then meditate profoundly on the white column (the Mental body) and will try to hear the still small voice, the subtle voice, the essence of INRI, the sibilant "S," the sharp sound of the crickets from the forests; thus, while making the effort of falling asleep profoundly, he will discard the Mental body by saying, "I am not the Mental body."

27. Now, the disciple will concentrate his entire mind on his willpower, and will discard the body of willpower by saying, "I am not willpower either."

28. Now let the disciple concentrate his mind on his consciousness, on Buddhi (body of the consciousness) and discard himself from that marvelous body by saying, "I am not the consciousness either."

29. Now let the disciple concentrate himself in his Innermost, become profoundly asleep, take a totally infantile attitude, and say, "I am the Innermost; I am the Innermost; I am the Innermost."

30. Let the disciple slumber even deeper and say, "The Innermost is just the child of the inner Christ."

31. Let the disciple profoundly meditate on the inner Christ.

32. Now the disciple should be absorbed within the inner Christ. Let the disciple be absorbed in Him, in Him, in Him.

33. Let the disciple say to himself, "I am He, I am He, I am He."

34. The mantra **Pander** will allow us to identify ourselves with our Inner Christ, so to act as Christ within the universe of Pleroma.

35. May the disciple become profoundly asleep, because sleep is the breach that allows us to pass from meditation into Samadhi.

36. There are many types of Samadhi: Astral Samadhi, Mental Samadhi,

Causal Samadhi, Samadhi within the consciousness, Samadhi within the Innermost, and Samadhi within the inner Christ.

37.   In the first Samadhi, we only enter into the Astral plane. We soar with the Mental body throughout space in the second type of Samadhi.

38.   We function without material vehicles of any type within the world of willpower in the third type of Samadhi. We soar with the Buddhic body throughout space in the fourth type of Samadhi.

39.   We can move in the Innermost without vehicles of any type throughout the World of the Mist of Fire in the fifth type of Samadhi.

40.   We can function in the inner Christ with the sixth type of Samadhi.

41.   There is a seventh type of Samadhi for the great Masters of Samadhi. In this Samadhi, we can visit the nucleoli upon which the entire universe is based. Those nucleoli, speaking in an allegorical way, are the holes through which we can observe the terrific majesty of the Absolute.

May the peace of the Father be with
ye.

Appendix
Shiva Samhita

Quoted by Samael Aun Weor in *The Perfect Matrimony,* and widely referred to by Hindu writers and mystics including Swami Sivananda, the mysterious text called *Shiva Samhita* ("Verses of Shiva") is a fractured, contradictory, and very misunderstood reference, especially among devotees of Hatha Yoga. Yet, when studied alongside other important Hindu texts, the genuine portions of the text become clearly obvious in contrast to the additions or corruptions.

Most of *Shiva Samhita* describes physical exercises originally designed to prepare the physical body for the more important work of sexual transmutation and meditation; of course, most readers of the text ignore this. We present here the most important section directly concerned with the sexual energy. As Samael Aun Weor said, we "leave the acrobatics to the circus performers." Gnosis is concerned with rapid spiritual awakening, thus we move directly to the point.

The text is written as though spoken by Shiva, the symbolic representative of the divine creative and destructive powers that we have within.

Vajroli-mudra

Actuated by mercy for my devotees, I [Shiva] shall now explain the Vajroli-mudra, the destroyer of the darkness of the world, the most secret among all secrets.

Even while living according to his wish and without conforming to the regulations of Yoga [i.e. remaining unmarried], a householder can become emancipated, if he practices the Vajroli-mudra.

This Vajroli yoga practice liberates even when immersed in his senses; therefore it should be practiced by the Yogi with great care [for without restraining the senses, it will lead to destruction].

First, according to the proper methods, let the wise yogi bring into his own body the generative power from the female organ of generation, by absorption through the phallus; restraining his semen, let him practice copulation [without orgasm].

When his sexual power is aroused, let him move his phallus [within the female organ]. If by chance the semen begins to move [out], let him stop its emission by the practice of the Yoni-mudra [restraint].

Let him withdraw the semen to the left [to be passive], and withdraw from intercourse. After a while, let him continue it again.

Following the guidance of his instructor and by uttering the sound hum, hum, let him absorb through the contraction of the Apana Vayu [wind energy; i.e pranayama] the creative elements of the yoni [feminine sexual organ].

By means of this practice, the Yogi, worshipper of the lotus-feet of his Guru, should obtain quick success in Yoga and drink celestial nectar [amrita, soma, ambrosia].

Know semen to be lunar [soma], and the seed is solar [Christic]; let the Yogi unite them in his body [through this practice].

I [Shiva] am the semen, Shakti [the Goddess] is the generative fluid; when they are [perfectly] combined in the body [through this practice], then the body of the Yogi becomes divine.

Ejaculation of semen brings death, preserving it within brings life. Therefore, one should make sure to retain the semen within.

One is born and dies through semen; in this there is no doubt. Knowing this, the Yogi must always preserve his semen.

When the precious jewel of semen is mastered, anything on earth can be mastered. Through the grace of its preservation, one becomes as great as me [Shiva].

The use of semen determines the happiness or pain of all beings living in the world, who are deluded [by desire] and are subject to death and decay.

This is the ultimate Yoga. Even though immersed in the world of the senses, one can reach perfection through its practice.

Without a doubt, through this practice the Yogi will acquire all kinds of powers, while at the same time enjoying the ecstasies of the world.

This Yoga can be practiced along with much enjoyment; therefore the Yogi should practice it.

[...]

I [Shiva] have revealed this Yoga because of love for my devotees. It should be guarded well [kept pure] with the greatest care, and not be given to everybody.

It is the most secret of all secrets that ever were or shall be [because misuse of it can create a demon]; therefore let the prudent Yogi guard it carefully [from becoming degenerated].

Glossary

Absolute: Abstract space; that which is without attributes or limitations. The Absolute has three aspects: the Ain, the Ain Soph, and the Ain Soph Aur.

"The Absolute is the Being of all Beings. The Absolute is that which Is, which always has Been, and which always will Be. The Absolute is expressed as Absolute Abstract Movement and Repose. The Absolute is the cause of Spirit and of Matter, but It is neither Spirit nor Matter. The Absolute is beyond the mind; the mind cannot understand It. Therefore, we have to intuitively understand Its nature." - Samael Aun Weor, *Tarot and Kabbalah*

"In the Absolute we go beyond karma and the gods, beyond the law. The mind and the individual consciousness are only good for mortifying our lives. In the Absolute we do not have an individual mind or individual consciousness; there, we are the unconditioned, free and absolutely happy Being. The Absolute is life free in its movement, without conditions, limitless, without the mortifying fear of the law, life beyond spirit and matter, beyond karma and suffering, beyond thought, word and action, beyond silence and sound, beyond forms."
- Samael Aun Weor, *The Major Mysteries*

Ahamkara: (Sanskrit, also ahankara) Egoism. The notion of the I as a self-existing, independent entity.

"The conception of "I," self-consciousness or self-identity; the "I," the egotistical and mayavic principle in man, due to our ignorance which seperates our "I" from the Universal One-self Personality, egoism." - The Theosophical Glossary.

Ahamkara is the existence of the ego, while *Ahamsara* is the dissolution of the "I."

"To truly eliminate the Ahamkara Bhava, the egoic condition from our consciousness, would be absolutely impossible if we commit the crime of forgetting our own Divine Mother Kundalini." - Samael Aun Weor, *The Gnostic Magic of the Runes*

Aryan Race: Quoted from Webster's Revised Unabridged Dictionary: "From Sanskrit [=a] rya excellent, honorable; akin to the name of the country Iran, and perh. to Erin, Ireland, and the early name of this people, at least in Asia. 1. One of a primitive people supposed to have lived in prehistoric times, in Central Asia, east of the Caspian Sea, and north of the Hindoo Koosh and Paropamisan Mountains, and to have been the stock from which sprang the Hindoo, Persian, Greek, Latin, Celtic, Teutonic, Slavonic, and other races; one of that ethnological division of mankind called also Indo-European or Indo-Germanic."

In Universal Gnosticism, this term refers to the vast majority of the popluation of this planet, and is noted for its close relationship with Ares or Mars, the God of War. Compare with "AquAryan" and "barbAryan." The Aryan race, the fifth great race to exist on this planet, is under the guidance of Ares, Mars, the Fifth of the "Seven Spirits before the Throne of God."

"Every Root Race has seven Subraces. The seed of our Aryan Root Race is Nordic, but when the Nordics mixed themselves with the Atlantean survivors, they gave origin onto the Subraces of the Aryan trunk.

"First Subrace: It flourished in central Asia, in those now vanished kingdoms of central Asia, and whose ruins still exist in the Himalayas around the country of Tibet. Powerful spiritual civilizations of the first Aryan Subrace existed in those regions.

"Second Subrace: It flourished in India and the entire south of Asia. In Pearland, the sacred land of the Vedas, in the ancient Hindustan, where the second Aryan Subrace developed, formidable esoteric cultures and tremendous civilizations existed.

"Third Subrace: It created powerful civilizations. Babylon, Chaldea, Egypt, etc., etc. were the scenario of very rich and powerful civilizations created by the third Aryan Subrace.

"Fourth Subrace: It developed in Rome, Greece, Italy, and Athens, the great city founded by the Goddess Athena. Before their degeneration and destruction, Greece and Italy were marvelous scenarios where the powerful civilizations of the fourth Aryan Subrace developed.

"Fifth Subrace: Are the Anglo-Saxon and Teutonic. The First and Second World Wars, with all of their barbarism and moral corruption, point with their accusatory fingers to the men and women of the fifth Aryan Subrace.

"Sixth Subrace: The mixture of the Spanish Conquistadors with the Native-American tribes. The effort to form the sixth Subrace in the redskin territory was very difficult, because the English Conquistadors destroyed them; they assassinated them, instead of mixing themselves with the natives. Only in a very insignificant and incipient way was the mixture of blood performed. This is why the Occult Fraternity saw the necessity of converting the North American territory into a melting crucible of races. So, the formation of the sixth Subrace in the United States had enormous difficulties; there, all the races of the world have mixed. The sixth Subrace in Latin America was formed very easily and this is something that must not be ignored by the treatisers of anthropogenesis and occultism.

"Seventh Subrace: The survivors of the new great cataclysm that soon will destroy this Aryan Root Race will be formed by the survivors of the Seventh Subrace; they do not exist yet, but they will.

"So, this Aryan Root Race, instead of evolving, has devolved, and its corruption is now worse than that of the Atlanteans in their epoch. Its wickedness is so great that it has reached unto heaven." - Samael Aun Weor, *The Kabbalah of the Mayan Mysteries*

Asana: (Sanskrit) Posture or position.

Bandha: Sanskrit term for "bondage" or "to bind together." Refers to postures in Hindu Yoga.

Bodhisattva: (Sanskrit; Tibetan: changchub sempa) Literally, Bodhi means "enlightenment" or "wisdom." Sattva means "essence" or "goodness," therefore the term Bodhisattva literally means "essence of wisdom." In the esoteric or secret teachings of Tibet and Gnosticism, a Bodhisattva is a human being who has reached the Fifth Initiation of Fire (Tiphereth) and has chosen to continue working by means of the Straight Path, renouncing the easier Spiral Path (in Nirvana), and returning instead to help suffering humanity. By means of this sacrifice, this individual incarnates the Christ (Avalokitesvara), thereby embodying the supreme source of wisdom and compassion. This is the entrance to the Direct Path to complete liberation from the ego, a route that only very few take, due to the fact that one must pay the entirety of one's karma in one life. Those who have taken this road have been the most remarkable figures in human history: Jesus, Buddha, Mohammed, Krishna, Moses, Padmasambhava, Milarepa, Joan of Arc, Fu-Ji, and many others whose names are not remembered or known. Of course, even among bodhisattvas there are many levels of Being: to be a bodhisattva does not mean that one is enlightened. Interestingly, the Christ in Hebrew is called Chokmah, which means "wisdom," and in Sanskrit the same is Vishnu, the root of the word "wisdom." It is Vishnu who sent his Avatars into the world in order to guide humanity. These avatars were Krishna, Buddha, Rama, and the Avatar of this age: the Avatar Kalki.

Brahmanadi: "The Brahmanadi or "canalis centralis" within which the Kundalini ascends exists throughout the length of the spinal medulla... Each one of our seven bodies has its own spinal medulla and its Brahmanadi." - Samael Aun Weor, *Kundalini Yoga*

"Within the Sushumna Nadi there is a Nadi by name Vajra. Chitra Nadi, a minute canal, which is also called Brahmanadi, is within this Vajra Nadi. Kundalini, when awakened, passes through Chitra Nadi." - Swami Sivananda, *Kundalini Yoga*

Brahmarandhra: (Sanskrit) "'Brahma-randhra' means the hole of Brahman. It is the dwelling house of the human soul. This is also known as "Dasamadvara," the tenth opening or the tenth door. The hollow place in the crown of the head known as anterior fontanelle in the new-born child is the Brahmarandhra. This is between the two parietal and occipital bones. This portion is very soft in a babe. When the child grows, it gets obliterated by the growth of the bones of the head. Brahma created the physical body and entered (Pravishat) the body to give illumination inside through this Brahmarandhra. In some of the Upanishads, it is stated like that. This is the most important part. It is very suitable for Nirguna Dhyana (abstract meditation). When the Yogi separates himself from the physical body at the time of death, this Brahmarandhra bursts open and Prana comes out through this opening (Kapala

Moksha). "A hundred and one are the nerves of
the heart. Of them one (Sushumna) has gone
out piercing the head; going up through it, one
attains immortality" (Kathopanishad)." - Swami
Sivananda, *Kundalini Yoga*

Buddhi: (Sanskrit, literally "intelligence") An
aspect of mind.

"Buddhi is pure [superior] reason. The seat of
Buddhi is just below the crown of the head in
the Pineal Gland of the brain. Buddhi is manifested only in those persons who have developed right intuitive discrimination or Viveka.
The ordinary reason of the worldly people is
termed practical reason, which is dense and has
limitations... Sankhya Buddhi or Buddhi in the
light of Sankhya philosophy is will and intellect
combined. Mind is microcosm. Mind is Maya.
Mind occupies an intermediate state between
Prakriti and Purusha, matter and Spirit." -
Swami Sivananda, *Yoga in Daily Life*

"When the diverse, confining sheaths of the
Atma have been dissolved by Sadhana, when
the different Vrittis of the mind have been
controlled by mental drill or gymnastic, when
the conscious mind is not active, you enter the
realm of spirit life, the super-conscious mind
where Buddhi and pure reason and intuition,
the faculty of direct cognition of Truth, manifest. You pass into the kingdom of peace where
there is none to speak, you will hear the voice
of God which is very clear and pure and has
an upward tendency. Listen to the voice with
attention and interest. It will guide you. It is

the voice of God." - Swami Sivananda, *Essence of Yoga*

In Kabbalah: The feminine Spiritual Soul, related to the sephirah Geburah. Symbolized throughout world literature, notably as Helen of Troy, Beatrice in The Divine Comedy, and Beth-sheba (Hebrew, literally "daughter of seven") in the Old Testament. The Divine or Spiritual Soul is the feminine soul of the Innermost (Atman), or his "daughter." All the strength, all the power of the Gods and Goddesses resides in Buddhi / Geburah, Cosmic Consciousness, as within a glass of alabaster where the flame of the Inner Being (Gedulah, Atman the Ineffable) is always burning.

Chaos: (Greek) There are three primary applications of this term.

"The first Chaos from which the cosmos emerged is between the Sephiroth Binah and Chesed. The second Chaos, from where the fundamental principles of the human being emerged, exists within Yesod-Mercury, which is the sexual human center. The third Chaos, the Infernal Worlds, exists below the Thirteenth Aeons in the region of Klipoth, in the underworld." - Samael Aun Weor, *The Gnostic Bible: The Pistis Sophia Unveiled*

The Abyss (not the Inferior Abyss), or the "Great Deep." Personified as the Egyptian Goddess Neith. The Great Mother, the Immaculate Virgin from which arises all matter. The Chaos is WITHIN the Ain Soph. The primitive state of the universe. Esoterically, a reference to the semen, both in the microcosm and the macrocosm. Alchemically, it is said to be a mixture of water & fire, and it holds the seeds of the cosmos.

Chakra: (Sanskrit) Literally, "wheel." The chakras are subtle centers of energetic transformation. There are hundreds of chakras in our hidden physiology, but seven primary ones related to the awakening of consciousness.

"The Chakras are centres of Shakti as vital force... The Chakras are not perceptible to the gross senses. Even if they were perceptible in the living body which they help to organise, they disappear with the disintegration of organism at death." - Swami Sivananda, *Kundalini Yoga*

"The chakras are points of connection through which the divine energy circulates from one to another vehicle of the human being." - Samael Aun Weor, *Aztec Christic Magic*

Christ: Derived from the Greek Christos, "the Anointed One," and Krestos, whose esoteric meaning is "fire." The word Christ is a title, not a personal name.

"Indeed, Christ is a Sephirothic Crown (Kether, Chokmah and Binah) of incommensurable wisdom, whose purest atoms shine within Chokmah, the world of the Ophanim. Christ is not the Monad, Christ is not the Theosophical Septenary; Christ is not the Jivan-Atman. Christ is the Central Sun. Christ is the ray that unites us to the Absolute." - Samael Aun Weor, *Tarot and Kabbalah*

Churches: The Christian symbol of the chakras or energetic centers.

Dharana: (Sanskrit) In Patanjali's Yoga, dharana is the fourth step, "concentration."

Dhyana: (Sanskrit; Tibetan sampten; Pali: jhana; Chinese: Ch'an; Japanese: zenna or zen) The Sanskrit term refers to "meditation," but is used to mean mental stability and active, meditative contemplation on the nature of an object.

1. In Hinduism, Dhyana is the fifth of the six stages of Patanjali's Yoga, and refers to state of conscious stillness, with perfect concentration on the object of meditation. From this, the sixth stage of Samadhi can be reached.

2. In Buddhism, Dhyana is the fifth of the six Paramitas (perfections). In Tibetan, the term sampten or bsam gtan means "definitive" or "established," because this is the basis from which all conscious realizations are reached.

Dhyani-pasa: (Sanskrit) "The rope of the Dhyanis or Spirits; the Pass-Not-Ring; the circle below which are all those who still labour under the delusion of seperateness." - The Theosophical Glossary.

Fohat: (Theosophical/Tibetan) A term used by H.P. Blavatsky to represent the active (male) potency of the Shakti (female sexual power) in nature, the essence of cosmic electricity, vital force. As explained in *The Secret Doctrine,* "He (Fohat) is, metaphysically, the objectivised thought of the gods; the "Word made flesh" on a lower scale, and the messenger of Cosmic and human ideations: the active force in Universal Life... In India, Fohat is connected with Vishnu and Surya in the early character of the (first) God;

for Vishnu is not a high god in the Rig Veda.
The name Vishnu is from the root vish, "to
pervade," and Fohat is called the "Pervader" and
the Manufacturer, because he shapes the atoms
from crude material..." The term fohat has
recently been linked with the Tibetan verb phro-
wa and the noun spros-pa. These two terms are
listed in Jäschke's Tibetan-English Dictionary
(1881) as, for phro-wa, "to proceed, issue, emanate from, to spread, in most cases from rays
of light..." while for spros-pa he gives "business,
employment, activity."

Gunas: (Sanskrit) Literally, "fundamental quality."

"Prakriti is composed of the three Gunas or
forces, namely, Sattva, Rajas and Tamas. Sattva
is harmony or light or wisdom or equilibrium
or goodness. Rajas is passion or motion or
activity. Tamas is inertia or inaction or darkness. During Cosmic Pralaya these three Gunas
exist in a state of equilibrium. During Srishti or
projection a vibration arises and the three quali-
ties are manifested in the physical universe."
- Swami Sivananda, *Kundalini Yoga*

"Sattva, Rajas and Tamas (harmony, emotion
and inertness) were in a perfect, nirvanic equilibrium before the dawning of the dawn of the
Mahamanvantara. The fire put the cosmic scale
in motion. Sattva, Rajas and Tamas were unbalanced; therefore, the Mahamanvantara dawned.
The yogi must liberate himself from Sattva,
Rajas and Tamas to gain the right to enter
into the Absolute. Sattva, Rajas and Tamas will
be in perfect equilibrium again at the end of
the Mahamanvantara; thus, the universe will

sleep again within the profound bosom of the Absolute, within the supreme Parabrahman, the Nameless." - Samael Aun Weor, *Kundalini Yoga*

Innermost: "Our real Being is of a universal nature. Our real Being is neither a kind of superior nor inferior "I." Our real Being is impersonal, universal, divine. He transcends every concept of "I," me, myself, ego, etc., etc." - Samael Aun Weor, *The Perfect Matrimony*

Also known as Atman, the Spirit, Chesed, our own individual interior divine Father.

"The Innermost is the ardent flame of Horeb. In accordance with Moses, the Innermost is the Ruach Elohim (the Spirit of God) who sowed the waters in the beginning of the world. He is the Sun King, our Divine Monad, the Alter-Ego of Cicerone." - Samael Aun Weor, *The Revolution of Beelzebub*

Jiva: (Sanskrit) The principle of life. Life, as the Absolute; or the Monad; or Atman-Buddhi.

Jnana: (Sanskrit) From the root jna, "to know." Knowledge; wisdom.

Kali: (Sanskrit, "the black one") In the sacred Vedas, this name refers to one of the seven tongues of Agni, the god of fire. The meaning has since changed to refer to the goddess Kali, the consort of Shiva.

"In India, Kali the Divine Mother Kundalini is adored, but Kali in her black, fatal aspect is also adored. These are the two Marys, the white and the black. The two Serpents, the Serpent of Brass which healed the Israelites in the

wilderness and the Tempting Serpent of Eden."
- Samael Aun Weor, *The Perfect Matrimony*

Kalki Avatar: (Sanskrit) According to the prophesies of India, in his tenth and final incarnation Lord Vishnu will incarnate himself as the Avatar Kalki, who will come riding his white horse and with his blazing sword in his hands. At the end of Kali Yuga (the present eon) He will punish all evil doers in this world, destroy this world, and recreate a golden age again. As it says in the ancient *Vishnu Purana:*

> "When the practices taught by the Vedas and the institutes of law shall nearly have ceased, and the close of the Kali age shall be nigh, a portion of that Divine Being who exists of his own spiritual nature in the character of Brahma, and who is the beginning and the end and who comprehends all things shall descend upon the earth. He will be born as Kalki in the family of an eminent brahmin, of Sambhala village, endowed with the eight superhuman faculties. By his irresistible might, He will destroy all the barbarians and thieves, and all whose minds are devoted to iniquity. He will then reestablish righteousness upon earth, and the minds of those who live at the end of the Kali age shall be awakened and shall be as pellucid as crystal. The men who are thus changed by virtue of that peculiar time shall be as the seeds of human beings and shall give birth to a race who shall follow the laws of the Krita Age, the Age of Purity." - Vishnu Purana 4.24

This is the Buddha Maitreya of the Mahayana
Buddhists, Sosiosh of the Zoroastrians, and
"The Faithful and True" of the book of The
Revelations of St. John 19:

> "And I saw heaven opened, and behold a
> white horse; and he that sat upon him was
> called Faithful and True, and in righteous-
> ness he doth judge and make war. His eyes
> were as a flame of fire, and on his head were
> many crowns; and he had a name written,
> that no man knew, but he himself. And he
> was clothed with a vesture dipped in blood:
> and his name is called The Word of God. And
> the armies which were in heaven followed
> him upon white horses, clothed in fine linen,
> white and clean (without ego). And out of his
> mouth goeth a sharp sword (the Word, the
> knowledge), that with it he should smite the
> nations: and he shall rule them with a rod of
> iron (Iron is the metal of Mars, of Samael):
> and he treadeth the winepress of the fierce-
> ness and wrath of Almighty God. And he hath
> on his vesture and on his thigh (next to the
> phallus) a name written, KING OF KINGS,
> AND LORD OF LORDS."

Kanda: Quoted from *Kundalini Yoga* by Swami
Sivananda: "This is situated between the anus
and the root of the reproductory organ. It is
like the shape of an egg and is covered with
membranes. This is just above the Muladhara
Chakra. All the Nadis of the body spring
from this Kanda. It is in the junction where
Sushumna is connected with Muladhara
Chakra. The four petals of the Muladhara

Chakra are on the sides of this Kanda and
the junction is called Granthi-Sthana, where
the influence of Maya is very strong. In some
Upanishads you will find that Kanda is 9
digits above the genitals. Kanda is a centre of
the astral body from where Yoga Nadis, subtle
channels, spring and carry the Sukshma Prana
(vital energy) to the different parts of the body.
Corresponding to this centre, you have 'Cauda
equina' in the gross physical body. The spinal
cord extending from the brain to the end of the
vertebral column tapers off into a fine silken
thread. Before its termination it gives off innumerable fibres, crowded into a bunch of nerves.
This bunch of nerves is 'Cauda equina' in the
gross body. The astral centre of 'Cauda equina'
is Kanda."

Kundalini: "Kundalini, the serpent power or
mystic fire, is the primordial energy or Sakti
that lies dormant or sleeping in the Muladhara
Chakra, the centre of the body. It is called the
serpentine or annular power on account of
serpentine form. It is an electric fiery occult
power, the great pristine force which underlies
all organic and inorganic matter. Kundalini
is the cosmic power in individual bodies. It
is not a material force like electricity, magnetism, centripetal or centrifugal force. It is a
spiritual potential Sakti or cosmic power. In
reality it has no form. [...] O Divine Mother
Kundalini, the Divine Cosmic Energy that is
hidden in men! Thou art Kali, Durga, Adisakti,
Rajarajeswari, Tripurasundari, Maha-Lakshmi,
Maha-Sarasvati! Thou hast put on all these

names and forms. Thou hast manifested as
Prana, electricity, force, magnetism, cohesion,
gravitation in this universe. This whole universe
rests in Thy bosom. Crores of salutations unto
thee. O Mother of this world! Lead me on
to open the Sushumna Nadi and take Thee
along the Chakras to Sahasrara Chakra and to
merge myself in Thee and Thy consort, Lord
Siva. Kundalini Yoga is that Yoga which treats
of Kundalini Sakti, the six centres of spiritual
energy (Shat Chakras), the arousing of the
sleeping Kundalini Sakti and its union with
Lord Siva in Sahasrara Chakra, at the crown of
the head. This is an exact science. This is also
known as Laya Yoga. The six centres are pierced
(Chakra Bheda) by the passing of Kundalini
Sakti to the top of the head. 'Kundala' means
'coiled'. Her form is like a coiled serpent. Hence
the name Kundalini." - Swami Sivananda,
Kundalini Yoga

"Kundalini is a compound word: Kunda
reminds us of the abominable "Kundabuffer
organ," and lini is an Atlantean term meaning
termination. Kundalini means "the termination
of the abominable Kundabuffer organ." In this
case, it is imperative not to confuse Kundalini
with Kundabuffer." - Samael Aun Weor, *The
Great Rebellion*

These two forces, one positive and ascending,
and one negative and descending, are symbolized in the Bible in the book of Numbers (the
story of the Serpent of Brass). The Kundalini
is "The power of life."- from the Theosophical

Glossary. The Sexual Fire that is at the base of all life.

"The ascent of the Kundalini along the spinal cord is achieved very slowly in accordance with the merits of the heart. The fires of the heart control the miraculous development of the Sacred Serpent. Devi Kundalini is not something mechanical as many suppose; the Igneous Serpent is only awakened with genuine Love between husband and wife, and it will never rise up along the medullar canal of adulterers." -Samael Aun Weor, *The Mystery of the Golden Blossom*

"The decisive factor in the progress, development and evolution of the Kundalini is ethics." - Samael Aun Weor, *The Revolution of Beelzebub*

"Until not too long ago, the majority of spiritualists believed that on awakening the Kundalini, the latter instantaneously rose to the head and the initiate was automatically united with his Innermost or Internal God, instantly, and converted into Mahatma. How comfortable! How comfortably all these theosophists, Rosicrucians and spiritualists, etc., imagined High Initiation." - Samael Aun Weor, *The Zodiacal Course*

"There are seven bodies of the Being. Each body has its "cerebrospinal" nervous system, its medulla and Kundalini. Each body is a complete organism. There are, therefore, seven bodies, seven medullae and seven Kundalinis. The ascension of each of the seven Kundalinis is slow and difficult. Each canyon or vertebra represents determined occult powers and this is why the conquest of each canyon undergoes terrible tests." - Samael Aun Weor, *The Zodiacal Course*

Laya: Sanskrit meaning, "point of dissolution" Laya is from the Sanskrit root li, meaning "to dissolve," "to disintegrate," or "to vanish away."

"The point of matter where every differentiation has ceased." - Blavatsky, *The Secret Doctrine.*

Logos: (Greek) means Verb or Word. In Greek and Hebrew metaphysics, the unifying principle of the world. The Logos is the manifested deity of every nation and people; the outward expression or the effect of the cause which is ever concealed. (Speech is the "logos" of thought). The Logos has three aspects, known universally as the Trinity or Trimurti. The First Logos is the Father, Brahma. The Second Logos is the Son, Vishnu. The Third Logos is the Holy Spirit, Shiva. One who incarnates the Logos becomes a Logos.

"The Logos is not an individual. The Logos is an army of ineffable beings." - Samael Aun Weor, *Fundamental Notions of Endocrinology & Criminology*

Logoi: (plural of Logos) In this book, the seven Logoi refers to the seven cosmocreators (self-realized Beings) who organize and manage the ray of creation.

Mahakalpa: (Sanskrit) "The Great (maha) Age (kalpa)."

Maha-kundalini: (Sanskrit) Maha means great.

"From the Mahakundalini (Cosmic Energy) the universe has sprung. In Her Supreme Form She is at rest, coiled round and one (as Chidrupini) with the Siva-bindu. She is then at rest. She next uncoils Herself to manifest. Here the three coils of which the Kundalini Yoga speaks are the three Gunas and the three and a half coil are the Prakriti and its three Gunas, together with the Vikritis. Her 50 coils are the letters of the Alphabet. As she goes on uncoiling, the Tattvas and the Matrikas, the Mother of the Varnas, issue from Her. She is thus moving, and continues even after creation to move in the Tattvas so created. For, as they are born of movement, they continue to move. The whole world (Jagat), as the Sanskrit term implies, is moving. She thus continues creatively acting until She has evolved Prithvi, the last of the Tattvas. First She creates mind, and then matter. This latter becomes more and more dense." - Swami Sivananda, *Kundalini Yoga*

Mahamanvantara: (Sanskrit) "The Great Day." A period of universal activity, as opposed to a Mahapralaya, a cosmic night or period of rest.

"I was absorbed within the Absolute at the end of that Lunar Mahamanvantara, which endured 311,040,000,000,000 years, or, in other words, an age of Brahma." - Samael Aun Weor, *The Revolution of Beelzebub*

"Truthfully, the quantities of years assigned to a Cosmic Day are symbolic. The Cosmic Night arrives when the ingathering of the perfect souls is complete, which means, when the Cosmic Day is absolutely perfected." - Samael Aun Weor, *The Gnostic Bible: The Pistis Sophia Unveiled*

Mantra: (Sanskrit, literally "mind protection") A sacred word or sound. The use of sacred words and sounds is universal throughout all religions and mystical traditions, because the root of all creation is in the Great Breath or the Word, the Logos. "In the beginning was the Word..."

Maya: (Sanskrit, literally "not That," meaning appearance, illusion, deception) Can indicate 1) the illusory nature of existence, 2) the womb of the Divine Mother, or 3) the Divine Mother Herself.

Mudra: (Tibetan, phyag rgya) Literally "mystic seal." This term implies a wide variety of meanings.

1. Commonly, this term is used by Hatha Yoga enthusiasts to refer to a system of postures or positions.

2. The Buddhist "Mahamudra" means Great Seal and refers to the realization acquired through the Mahayana and Vajrayana paths.

3. In Vajrayana Buddhism, the mudra is the female consort or partner in the practice of Karmamudra (sexual magic).

4. Asian art depicts gods and goddesses displaying a variety of hand positions, called mudras.

5. In the five "M's" of the Pancatattva Ritual (also called panchamakara), mudra refers to grain.

Nadi: (Sanskrit; Tibetan tsa) Nerve channel for subtle energies. "The term Nadi comes from the root Nad which means motion. The body is filled with an uncountable number of Nadis. If they were revealed to the eye, the body would present the appearance of a highly-complicated chart of ocean currents. Superficially the water seems one and the same. But examination shows that it is moving with varying degrees of force in all directions." - Swami Sivananda, *Kundalini Yoga*

Parabrahman: (Sanskrit, literally "the highest brahman") The Absolute or universal self.

Paramarthasatya: (Sanskrit) Para, "absolute, supreme." Parama, "that which knows, or the consciousness." Artha, "that which is known." Satya, "existence, Truth." In synthesis, "The supreme knowledge of all that exists: TRUTH."

1) A being of very high development; an inhabitant of the Absolute.

2) The ultimate truth, as opposed to conventional truth (samvriti-satya) or relative truth of the manifested world.

Pleroma: (Greek) "Fullness," an ancient Gnostic term adopted to signify the divine world or Universal Soul. Space, developed and divided into a series of aeons. The abode of the invisible Gods. In correspondence to the Kabbalah, Pleroma refers to the World of Atziluth.

Prajapati: (Sanskrit, literally "lord of creatures") A title in the *Vedas* referring to Indra. In general, it refers to any divinity who creates life.

There are said to be children of Indra (Gods) who create life as well. In Gnosis, the prajapatis usually referred to are the Elohim or the "seven spirits before the throne": the seven cosmocreators who sustain life in a given solar system.

"Progenitors; the givers of life to all on this earth. They are seven and ten - corresponding to the seven and ten Kabbalistic Sephiroth; to the Mazdean Amesha-Spentas, etc." - The Theosophical Glossary.

Prana: (Sanskrit; Tibetan bindu) Life-principle; the breath of life; energy. The vital breath, which sustains life in a physical body; the primal energy or force, of which other physical forces are manifestations. In the books of Yoga, prana is described as having five modifications, according to its five different functions. These are: prana (the vital energy that controls the breath), apana (the vital energy that carries downward unassimilated food and drink), samana (the vital energy that carries nutrition all over the body), vyama (the vital energy that pervades the entire body), and udana (the vital energy by which the contents of the stomach are ejected through the mouth). The word Prana is also used as a name of the Cosmic Soul, endowed with activity.

Pranayama: (Sanskrit for "restraint (ayama) of prana (energy, life force)") A type of breathing exercise that transforms the life force (sexual energy) of the practitioner.

"Pranayama is a system of sexual transmutation for single persons." - Samael Aun Weor, *The Yellow Book*

Pranava: (Sanskrit) A sacred word.

Purusha: (Sanskrit) Supreme being.

"Behind this world show, behind this physical phenomena, behind these names and forms, behind the feelings, thoughts, emotions, sentiments, there dwells the silent witness, thy immortal Friend and real Well-wisher, the Purusha or the World-teacher, the invisible Power or Consciousness." - Swami Sivananda, *God Exists*

"That secondless Supreme Being, who resides in the chambers of your heart as the Inner Ruler or Controller, who has no beginning, middle or end, is God or Atman, or Brahman or Purusha or Chaitanya or Bhagavan or Purushottama." - Swami Sivananda

Sadhaka: (Sanskrit) Spiritual aspirant.

Samadhi: (Sanskrit) Literally means "union" or "combination" and its Tibetan equivilent means "adhering to that which is profound and definitive," or ting nge dzin, meaning "To hold unwaveringly, so there is no movement." Related terms include satori, ecstasy, manteia, etc. Samadhi is a state of consciousness. In the west, the term is used to describe an ecstatic state of consciousness in which the Essence escapes the painful limitations of the mind (the "I") and therefore experiences what is real: the Being, the Great Reality. There are many levels of Samadhi. In the sutras and tantras the term Samadhi has a much broader application whose precise interpretation depends upon which school and teaching is using it.

"Ecstasy is not a nebulous state, but a transcendental state of wonderment, which is associated with perfect mental clarity." - Samael Aun Weor, *The Elimination of Satan's Tail*

Sannyasin: (Sanskrit, literally "he who has cast aside") A renunciate.

Serpents of Fire: The Initiations of Major Mysteries, which are the beginning stages of the First Mountain, the Mountain of Initiation. Through the accomplishment of these processes, the initiate creates the Solar Bodies. For details, read *The Perfect Matrimony* and *The Three Mountains*.

Serpents of Light: Any initiate who completes the Serpents of Fire AND chooses to continue by walking on the Direct Path then enters into the second half of the First Mountain. The Christ is born inside the initiate, who then begins to illuminate each of the seven bodies of the soul (the spinal column of each body is filled with the Light of the Christ).

Sexual Magic: The word magic is derived from the ancient word magos "one of the members of the learned and priestly class," from O.Pers. magush, possibly from PIE *magh- "to be able, to have power." [Quoted from Online Etymology Dictionary].

"All of us possess some electrical and magnetic forces within, and, just like a magnet, we exert a force of attraction and repulsion... Between lovers that magnetic force is particularly powerful and its action has a far-reaching effect."
- Samael Aun Weor, *The Mystery of the Golden Blossom*

Sexual magic refers to an ancient science that has been known and protected by the purest, most spiritually advanced human beings, whose purpose and goal is the harnessing and perfection of our sexual forces. A more accurate translation of sexual magic would be "sexual priesthood." In ancient times, the priest was always accompanied by a priestess, for they represent the divine forces at the base of all creation: the masculine and feminine, the Yab-Yum, Ying-Yang, Father-Mother: the Elohim. Unfortunately, the term "sexual magic" has been grossly misinterpreted by mistaken persons such as Aleister Crowley, who advocated a host of degenerated practices, all of which belong solely to the lowest and most perverse mentality and lead only to the enslave-ment of the consciousness, the worship of lust and desire, and the decay of humanity. True, upright, heavenly sexual magic is the natural harnessing of our latent forces, making them active and harmonious with nature and the divine, and which leads to the perfection of the human being.

"People are filled with horror when they hear about sexual magic; however, they are not filled with horror when they give themselves to all kinds of sexual perversion and to all kinds of carnal passion." - Samael Aun Weor, *The Perfect Matrimony*

Shiva: A multifacted symbol in the Hindu pan-theon.

"Lord Siva is the pure, changeless, attributeless, all-pervading transcendental consciousness.... At the end of Pralaya, the Supreme Lord thinks of re-creation of the world. He is then known by the name Sadasiva. He is the root-cause

of creation. From Sadasiva creation begins...
[Additionally,] Lord Siva represents the destructive aspect of Brahman... He destroys all bondage, limitation and sorrow of His devotees. He
is the giver of Mukti or the final emancipation.
He is the universal Self. He is the true Self of all
creatures. He is the dweller in the cremation-
ground, in the region of the dead, those who
are dead to the world. The Jivas and the world
originate from Him, exist in Him, are sustained
and rejected by Him and are ultimately merged
in Him. He is the support, source and substra-
tum of the whole world. He is an embodiment
of Truth, Beauty, Goodness and Bliss. He is
Satyam, Sivam, Subham, Sundaram, Kantam.
He is the God of gods, Deva-Deva. He is the
Great Deity—Mahadeva." - Swami Sivananda,
Lord Siva and His Worship

The Hindu Creator and Destroyer, the third
aspect of the Trimurti (Brahma, Vishnu, Shiva).
The Third Logos. The Holy Spirit. The Sexual
Force. The Sephira Binah. Symbolized by a
Linga / lingum, a male sexual organ.

Sushumna: "When we study the construction,
location and function of the Spinal Cord and
the Sushumna Nadi, we can readily say that
the Spinal Cord was called Sushumna Nadi by
the Yogins of yore. The Western Anatomy deals
with the gross form and functions of the Spinal
Cord, while the Yogins of ancient times dealt
with all about the subtle (Sukshma) nature.
Now in Kundalini Yoga, you should have a
thorough knowledge of this Nadi. Sushumna
extends from the Muladhara Chakra (second

vertebra of coccygeal region) to Brahmarandhra.
The Western Anatomy admits that there is a
central canal in the Spinal Cord, called Canalis
Centralis and that the cord is made up of grey
and white brain-matter. Spinal Cord is dropped
or suspended in the hollow of the spinal column. In the same way, Sushumna is dropped
within the spinal canal and has subtle sections."
- Swami Sivananda, *Kundalini Yoga*

Tattva: (Sanskrit) "truth, fundamental principle."
A reference to the essential nature of a given
thing. Tattvas are the elemental forces of
nature. There are numerous systems presenting
varying tattvas as fundamental principles of
nature. Gnosticism utilizes a primary system
of five: akash (which is the elemental force of
the ether), tejas (fire), vayu (air), apas (water)
and prittvi (earth). Two higher tattvas are also
important: adi and samadhi.

White Brotherhood: That ancient collection
of pure souls who maintain the highest and
most sacred of sciences: White Magic or White
Tantrism. It is called White due to its purity
and cleanliness. This "Brotherhood" or "Lodge"
includes human beings of the highest order
from every race, culture, creed and religion, and
of both sexes.

Yoga: (Sanskrit) "union." Similar to the Latin
"religare," the root of the word "religion." In
Tibetan, it is "rnal-'byor" which means "union
with the fundamental nature of reality."

"The word YOGA comes from the root Yuj
which means to join, and in its spiritual sense,
it is that process by which the human spirit is

brought into near and conscious communion with, or is merged in, the Divine Spirit, according as the nature of the human spirit is held to be separate from (Dvaita, Visishtadvaita) or one with (Advaita) the Divine Spirit." - Swami Sivananda, *Kundalini Yoga*

"The word 'yoga' means in general to join one's mind with an actual fact..." - The 14th Dalai Lama

"The soul aspires for the union with his Innermost, and the Innermost aspires for the union with his Glorian." - Samael Aun Weor, *The Revolution of Beelzebub*

"All of the seven schools of Yoga are within Gnosis, yet they are in a synthesized and absolutely practical way. There is Tantric Hatha Yoga in the practices of the Maithuna (Sexual Magic). There is practical Raja Yoga in the work with the chakras. There is Gnana Yoga in our practices and mental disciplines which we have cultivated in secrecy for millions of years. We have Bhakti Yoga in our prayers and rituals. We have Laya Yoga in our meditation and respiratory exercises. Samadhi exists in our practices with the Maithuna and during our deep meditations. We live the path of Karma Yoga in our upright actions, in our upright thoughts, in our upright feelings, etc." - Samael Aun Weor, *The Revolution of Beelzebub*

"The Yoga that we require today is actually ancient Gnostic Christian Yoga, which absolutely rejects the idea of Hatha Yoga. We do not recommend Hatha Yoga simply because, spiritually speaking, the acrobatics of this discipline are fruitless; they should be left to the acrobats of the circus." - Samael Aun Weor, *The Yellow Book*

Yogi: (Sanskrit) male yoga practitioner.

Yogini: (Sanskrit) female yoga practitioner.

Index

Glorian Publishing is a non-profit publisher dedicated to spreading the sacred universal doctrine to suffering humanity. All of our works are made possible by the kindness and generosity of sponsors. If you would like to make a tax-deductible donation, you may send it to the address below, or visit our website for other alternatives. If you would like to sponsor the publication of a book, please contact us at 877-726-2359 or help@gnosticteachings.org.

Glorian Publishing
PO Box 110225
Brooklyn, NY 11211 US
Phone: 877-726-2359

VISIT US ONLINE AT:

gnosticteachings.org